ANTI-AGING

Natural Remedies and Practices to Prevent Aging

(Anti-aging by Achieving Your Optimum Health
With Nutrition Balance)

Horace Rhodes

Published By Zoe Lawson

Horace Rhodes

All Rights Reserved

Anti-aging: Natural Remedies and Practices to Prevent Aging (Anti-aging by Achieving Your Optimum Health With Nutrition Balance)

ISBN 978-1-77485-255-2

Legal & Disclaimer

The information contained in this book is not designed to replace or take the place of any form of medicine or professional medical advice. The information in this book has been provided for educational and entertainment purposes only.

The information contained in this book has been compiled from sources deemed reliable, and it is accurate to the best of the Author's knowledge; however, the Author cannot guarantee its accuracy and validity and cannot be held liable for any errors or omissions. Changes are periodically made to this book. You must consult your doctor or get professional medical advice before using any of the suggested remedies, techniques, or information in this book.

TABLE OF CONTENTS

Introduction

We live in a time of innovation and technology, technologies that have made our lives effortless, quick and speedy. While it is many benefits our modern lifestyle is also bringing a host of challenges. Due to the rising pollution of the air and the rapid pace of life, it's been difficult to monitor our physical health as well as mental health. Everyone wants to appear young and beautiful for the rest of their lives. However, because of pollution in the air the goal has become extremely difficult to attain.

Humans have been fascinated by the idea of eternal youth and immortality ever since the time. Everyone wants to live for as long as they can and keep their body and skin in good shape and health. Our mythologies are full of stories and legends about people who have lost their lives in search to attain immortality. For example, the myths about The Fountain of Youth.

However, we've looked to find the Fountain from the wrong spots. It is, in reality all around us!

Nature is the real Fountain of Youth. It's unfortunate that we are still struggling to discover the mysteries of nature, and aren't able to comprehend it fully. That's why we don't realize the wealth of nature, and why we not be able to solve the issues. But instead of focusing on ways to tackle these issues, we should instead focus on other blessings nature could give us. One of these gifts is, obviously the young.

There are many natural ingredients which can be used to keep looking healthy and young for a long period of time. This book contains a compilation of recipes and ingredients that can be used to attain the Fountain of Youth, that is without any adverse consequences!

Within this publication, you'll discover simple and healthy recipes to help you attain an attractive and youthful skin. There are a range of packs, concoctions and lotions. made from 100% natural ingredients that can boost the glow of your skin and help your body and skin appear younger for longer. This is all without adverse consequences! So, continue reading to find out how you can find the secret to remaining young for all time.

Chapter 1: How and Why Does It Happen

The first step towards battling the aging process is to know the definition of aging, and the reasons why it occurs. We all are aware that our bodies alter when we get older. We can gaze at ourselves in the mirror and notice lines and wrinkles. Many treatments focus on wrinkles but fail to consider that they are simply the visible evidence of an internal process.

As we get older the cells of our skin undergo significant changes. The human skin is composed of three layers. The outermost layer - the one that causes wrinkles is called the epidermis. The skin cells we see at the mirror are actually dead hardened cells that shield our bodies from elements and damage. Below that is the dermis, which is responsible for collagen and elastin, two chemical compounds that keep our skin healthy and elastic. The lower layer is known as the hypodermis. It is composed of fat.

The body sheds hundreds of cells each day. Cells that are dying die and fall off, while new cells appear to fill in their place. As the body ages the process slows. The process takes longer eliminate dead cells and it can take longer for the body to create new cells. In the dermis collagen, its distribution is erratic while the process of production decreases. In this case the epidermis shrinks or wrinkles. the appearance is dull.

The image on left shows the epidermis that is smooth, as well as the dermis underneath and its evenly distributed collagen fibers. As we age the dermis is able to produce large quantities of collagen. The collagen fibers have a uniform distribution across the dermis, giving the epidermis the smooth look typical of youthfulness. As we age as we age, the dermis produces less collagen, and its distribution become irregular, as you observe in the image to the right. The decreased collagen and uneven distribution of it across the dermis can cause wrinkles and sagging of the epidermis.

There are many other signs of aging, beyond wrinkles. A different symptom that is visible is age spots. These are also visible in the picture to the right. Unintentional exposure to sun is the main cause of age spots as well as exposure to UV radiation during the wrong time can increase the aging process of the dermis, just as is smoking.

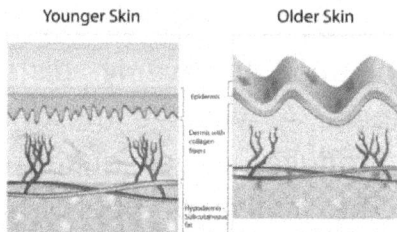

Younger Skin   Older Skin

It is essential that you get exposure to the sunlight. Sunlight is the most secure and source for Vitamin D. But the best times to get sun exposure are in the morning prior to 10 am and in the afternoon, between 3-4 after 3-4 pm. Averaging 20-30 minutes per day is an adequate quantity of sun exposure. In addition, by eating a balanced diet high in antioxidants, and having plenty of vegetables and fruits, your capacity to heal from sunburn or skin damage is increased.

Systemic Age-related Signs

Age spots and wrinkles are not the only external manifestations of the aging process. As we age our bodies undergo a transformation. The cells get bigger, and are slower to divide and grow. The connective tissues become stiffer and lose flexibility which causes the usual discomforts and aches that accompany aging. In more serious instances joints may stiffen up to the point that they can hinder normal activities. As we age, conditions such as arthritis are becoming more frequent. One reason is that connective tissues such as cartilage have a limited capacity for regenerative power which makes them more vulnerable to the signs of getting older. Research has demonstrated the link with animal products and other harmful food items in our diet to the development of arthritis.

Furthermore, changes in cell membranes can make it difficult for cells to absorb their nutrients and oxygen they require. Some cells show increased pigmentation and start to store the toxins and fats. The damage is permanent to certain types of cells, which do not regenerate in any way like the heart and muscles, nerves and the lens of our eyes.

Internal organs are slow in their work too. As we grow older heart organs can pump ten many times more blood that our bodies require. At the age of 30 it is estimated that we lose around one percent of that capacity every year. Also, we lose function in our kidneys, lungs and liver, though this amount may vary dependent on other factors, such as your genetics as well as personal habits such as drinking or smoking. External stressors can cause the deficiency of organs also.

A different side effect of aging is the loss of metabolism. Metabolism is a process that our bodies employ to process food that we consume. As metabolism decreases, we the body burns less calories and could increase weight. Being overweight, obviously, adds pressure on our body overall. For instance arthritis and joint pain are made worse when we carry additional weight. Additionally, the extra weight adds additional strain on our hearts as well as other organs within us.

Aging isn't just a one-time process. Instead, it's an intricate set of factors and shifts. Certain of these changes are expected but others can be seen or increase due to the ways we live our lives. We're usually so eager to slow the signs of ageing that we don't consider what causes these symptoms. And, even more importantly, we tackle the symptoms using radical treatments that involve extreme chemicals or even surgery, but ignore the fact that treatments often cause more harm than the signs. It's time to begin looking at the particular processes that lead to ageing and ways to alter them from the inside out.

Chapter 2: Preventive Measures is Possible

Therefore, rather than bombarding you with all the research in one go This chapter is devoted to offering simple solutions, along with a few of them explained in greater details. This chapter focuses on getting the ball rolling in a way (no joke intended) and offering an easy-to-follow but effective strategies on how to deal with the more unpleasant symptoms of ageing.

* Drink green tea

• Resistance training- If you're worried about the decrease of skin elasticity that occurs with age and may result in things like ugly bat wings, do not fret there are ways to minimize or even stop the appearance of these wings. Resistance training is among the methods. Experts recommend about forty-five minutes of training in resistance every week, three times per week for the most effective results. Therefore, the next time you workout or are searching for new equipment for your workout consider buying a resistance band or similar equipment.

* Consume grapefruit- vitamin C, either 75 mg or more per day is proven to lessen wrinkles

* Make use of apple cider vinegar as a toner

* Reduce your sugar intake

Avoid high heels- the practice of walking or standing in heels for prolonged and extended periods of time is known to increase the chance to develop varicose veins. If you're contemplating one of your top outfits, you might want to put off the pumps and opt to a pair of fashionable flats instead.

* Make use of coconut oil as a moisturizer

* Take a bite of Brazil nuts. They are known for their selenium content, Brazil nuts can help fight UV damage

Eat a lot of berries. We all are aware that berries contain antioxidants and give us a plethora of health benefits. But what we may not realize is that they are especially beneficial in the fight against aging as they contain anthocyanins that are believed to fight and slow the progression of certain cancers, boost and improve the functioning of the brain, and increasing the amount of muscle tone lost as we the passage of time.

Smile an exercise- there are numerous exercises that require a lot of smiling and relaxation to tone the skin in order to fight the sagging cheeks and cheeks.

* Drink plenty of water, and plenty of it.

* Toothpaste! In order to rid yourself of the yellow marks that are under the nails of yours, you can try rubbing the nail with a bit of toothpaste to whiten your teeth.

Do a workout! Exercises that are high in cardio will ensure you get sufficient oxygen and essential nutrients to your skin to fight the age-related signs

* Yoga - the stretching, conditioning and general relaxation that come through yoga can help improve the appearance of skin and avoid wrinkles caused by stress.

Try a cleanse Many of the foods we take into our bodies contain toxins and other harmful substances. Whatever your cleanse is a short, fast juice-based diet or eliminating carbohydrates from your diet Try it. This short break will allow your body and skin the chance to recover and balance out. Make sure to speak with your physician prior to beginning any treatment to make sure you're still getting the nutrients you require.

* Black tea- If you're worried about plaque formation and yellowing drinking black tea is recognized to fight these undesirable negative effects.

* Floss!

Eat a large amount of tomatoes The tomatoes contain lycopene an antioxidant that can help reduce the risk of some cancers and also maintain youthful looking skin and smooth skin.

* Take a bite of dark chocolate

Take a sip of Joe* Sip a cup of Joe Swedish as well as Finnish researchers have discovered the consumption of coffee about 3-4 cups per day has been proven to decrease the risk of developing dementia by as much as 65 percent. Just make sure that you don't drink after 3 pm to can rest.

Be aware of your weight And remember, when even though we're saying manage, this does not mean you have to go insane! Consult your doctor first.

* Sleep- It's difficult to imagine how this simple thing can be so beneficial, but it can be! Sleeping in a sufficient amountthat last longer than 6 hours per night - can reduce stress levels overall and also help lower the risk of developing heart disease.

Take your leafy dark greens

If you sleep on your back,It is the American Academy of Dermatology has found that those who lie on their backs are more prone to wrinkles because of the etching lines left by our bed which don't disappear when we wake up. If you've no preference for your sleep and are equally comfortable to sleep in your back position, you should make the change!

* Eat fish! Particularly, fish that is rich in omega-3s and fatty acids helps reduce inflammation, improve mood and reduce risk of developing heart disease.

* Strengthen your muscles!

* Don't look at the screen.

* Berries! In general, anything that is packed with antioxidants is great for aiding in the fight against aging.

* Take red wine in moderation

* Laugh often, and frequently.

• Take your vitamins! Vitamins, especially C, E and A, give us antioxidants to fight off the less desirable aspects of aging and are also good food items for any healthy diet.

* Pat your face dry, don't rub it.

Use your ring finger, If you do apply moisturizing use your ring finger because it's the most weak finger and less likely apply pressure too strongly and leave marks that don't look good.

Eat your veggies and fruits!

Increase your mood studies have proven that the more content you are, the younger you appear. Although it appears to be a bit simple, there is science backing this up!

* Laugh frequently

* Use mild, fragrance-free soap. soap.

It's nap time! Everyday, take an easy, but rejuvenating 30 minute nap.

We've now taken some time to provide some tips and tricks and tricks, let's get to something beyond simple prevention.

Chapter 3: Food To Add To Your Diet To Help Fight Skin Aging

What to Eat

The skin must be taken care of and protected to minimize the signs of the aging process. One way to take care of your skin is by eating a healthy diet and consuming a nutritious diet. We hear these words often What exactly is a good nutrition and diet mean?

A diet that is rich in nutrients which protect skin from damage from free radicals is the ideal diet. Foods high with vitamins A C E, and zinc aid in stimulating the renewal of skin cells and improve overall health of the skin. Foods that are rich in antioxidants help fight free radicals that damage the cells of the skin.

Here are some food items you could consider adding to your diet.

The skin of grapes is the resveratrol, a potent antioxidant that fights premature ageing. Resveratrol is an anti-inflammatory too. A diet that involves eating grapes or drinking a glasses of wine every day is a great way to combat the signs of ageing. Make sure you don't consume at least one glass of wine per day as drinking too much isn't good for your body. If alcohol isn't your style, then drink wine instead.

Berries-Blueberries, raspberries and strawberries are all fruits that have high levels of antioxidants that combat free radicals. These fruits also come packed with vitamin C, which helps keep your skin looking youthful. Vitamin C high-quality foods like strawberries can help fight wrinkles and dryness.

Oats can be a an ingredient for your skin, or as a scrub to get rid of those dead cells to reveal fresh skin. Oats have a low glycemic index, which means it reduces cholesterol levels and increases the risk of diabetes. Foods high in glycemic index cause wrinkles to appear on the face.

Whole Grains: Brown barley, wheat, rice Oats, quinoa, and quinoa include all grains high in fiber. A diet that is rich in fiber helps keep blood vessels in good condition so that blood can circulate efficiently through the whole body. When blood flows through the body freely, it is able to efficiently oxygenate cells so that they can regenerate themselves. This will give you a smoother skin.

Citrus Fruits Vitamin C is a vital vitamin that aids the body to fight off illness and keeps your body healthy. Vitamin C helps keep the cell walls of the skin healthy through fighting free radicals which can damage the cells. Vitamin C also promotes creation of collagen. Lemons, oranges, kiwis and grapefruits are all rich in large amounts of vitamin C.

Vegetables - Vegetables are rich in many minerals and vitamins vital to collagen production and cell renewal in the skin. Vitamin A boosts cell turnover and stimulates the growth of skin cell growth.

Try Brussel sprouts and kale as well as spinach to help keep your skin firm.

Protein rich foods such as lean foods like legumes, meat, and even fish are the best proteins. Collagen is made of protein. Therefore, eating proteins rich foods can assist in the creation of collagen. Protein-rich foods can also be muscles builders. Be sure to not cook meats until they have been charcoal-grilled. Charred meat may contain cancer-causing chemicals.

The carrots and the tomatoes are rich in Lycopene as well as beta-carotene. Both protect you against harmful UV radiations. Research has shown that those who eat food that is with high levels of beta-carotene and lycopene tend to be less likely be sunburned compared to those who don't. It is still necessary to apply sunblock, even if you consume these food items. Carrots are also rich in vitamin A that aids in maintaining the health of the scalp. A healthy scalp means healthy, shiny, youthful hair.

Fish- Fish, such as salmon are rich of Omega 3 fatty acids. Omega 3 fights damage caused by UV radiation and makes the skin appear more soft and smooth. It also increases skin elasticity and ensures that skin cells are healthy. Fish, such as cod, are rich in selenium, which assists in keeping skin healthy and free of damage and cancer caused by harmful UV Rays. Include the wild fish like tuna, and Sardines to the diet of your choice at least three every week.

Foods that are rich in Monosaturated FatsAvocadoes, as well as olive oil are two of the food items that are high in monosaturated or monosaturated oils. They are full of biotin that promotes healthy skin. Monosaturated fats are healthy fats that help keep skin cells healthy.

Dark Chocolate -Dark chocolates also contain the resveratrol. Dark chocolate is also high in flavonoids, which can assist in fighting free radicals. Consume 70% cocoa in order to get the most benefit in dark cocoa. Avoid sweeter varieties since they could contain very little cacao content, and may contain more sugar.

Nuts-Almondsand walnuts, Pistachios and other nuts are high in vitamin E that aids in the regeneration in skin cell renewal. Vitamin E helps to protect the skin from harmful UV rays, too. In lieu of reaching for the box of chips opt for some nuts. They'll provide more energy and fiber over that salty snack.

Water - Water hydrates skin cells in the same way as any other part within the body. Water aids in promoting good blood circulation, too. Take 8 glass of fluids every daily to ensure that you're properly hydrated. Water is also a great way to flush out toxic substances in your body.

Which Foods Not to Eat

They are likely the food items that you consume on a regular basis. Reduce your intake of these food items if they are included in your diet, as they're not only harmful to your skin. But can be harmful to your overall health.

Sugar-Sugar content in processed food items, cakes and candy causes wrinkles and dull skin. Foods with a sugar in high amounts damage the collagen and elastin within the skin. There is always a sugar in their lives, so sugar can't be completely eliminated. Cut down on your sugar consumption by substituting honey to sweeten your tea or choose black coffee instead of adding sugar in it.

White Bread and Pasta- These contain high levels of glycemic, which are, as we have mentioned are food items that cause wrinkles and can also cause the appearance of acne in some instances.

SaltSalt causes swelling and makes your face appear puffy. It holds water and makes that you appear like you're bloated. Salt causes puffiness , particularly around the eyes that makes you appear more noticeable. It can also increase the risk of having high blood pressure.

Alcohol Consumption: Alcohol is detrimental to your body. It's harmful to the skin since it dehydrates the skin and makes it dull and dry. The body attempts to compensate for the dehydration through taking your reserves. A majority of them are taken from the skin.

Processed foods are laden with preservatives and chemicals that are detrimental to your body. These chemicals can cause harm to the body's cells, such as skin cells. Foods processed for processing are loaded with sodium and sugar, and also. Be sure to stay away from processed food in the maximum extent you can.

Chapter 4: The Art of Fine Tuning Your Mental Persistence Everyday

How do you begin? Consider starting with the mind? Seeing as the mind is the leader and the body follows. If you are able to keep your brain in check and your mind agile, then you'll be able to live your life to some capacity, and retain your dignity. The best part is that a well-balanced mind will assist in giving you a healthier and stronger body. Your mind is the one that controls the movements of your body, and that is the most important factor to maintaining a healthy biomechanics and muscle control.

Let's look at the problems you could face in this area as you get older and ways to keep the issues at low...

Cognitive Decline As We Age

The most common thing we identify with cognitive decline due to age is the tendency to forget. As you get to an age at which you begin to forget where you put your keys a bit more frequently, and then you begin to forget the names of your family members. Call everyone Frank It's much more convenient.

A small amount of loss of memory is quite normal with age , and is often referred to as "age-related cognitive decline'. However, in certain instances it may lead to a more severe type of dementia known as Alzheimer's disease. This results from amyloid plaques as well as neurofibrillary tangles. They result from a build-up of protein fragments attached to cells.

This may cause confusion and memory loss, known as Alzheimer's or dementia. In certain cases the loss of memory and confusion are caused by brain damage that is caused by strokes or trauma to the brain.

But before that, is the slight fatigue and brain fog. It's not noticeable, but it's certain to be there. As with a computer which needs an extra few minutes to get up and running. Nobody else will notice and you'll know that it's not firing at full speed any more. Not as it was.

Take a moment to think about how much more difficult is it to get to the world in the early morning as in the last five years? In the past, you'd likely have been out drinking all night with your friends, only to you would wake up the next day with a jolt of energy. Your body isn't altered at the moment the brain is at fault...

What about thinking about going back further (memory by allowing ...) to) back when you were a young child. In the past, you could go about in circles and circles for hours without exhausting yourself. You probably know children who perform the same activity.

Today, however, a lot of us struggle to climb the staircase!

Tiredness isn't enjoyment, and neither is only half the enthusiasm you did in your younger years or the capacity or enthusiasm to learn. Take note of how youngsters are constantly learning new things while making new friends, as well as changing careers. This is harder as you get older.

And what is your attitude? Are you aware that you're feeling more angry constantly these days? Things that once would have given us to think about it today has us grumbling in our breaths like crazy people. What has happened to the youthful optimism? If you're familiar with the 'law of attraction', then you'll be aware of how constantly angry can result in fewer chances and less fun. Evidently, it's when you reach an age that's 60 that these changes take place.

What's happening in your cranium that's causing this transformation?

Enhancing Mood and Brain Energy Through Nutrition and Nootropics

There are a myriad of things that alter the brain and are responsible for the changes that we notice in our capabilities and personality. Some of these changes can be mitigated with the proper nutrient and/or supplement regimen however when supplements, herbs, or medicines are utilized in this manner, they're often called "nootropics," which are substances which can aid in improving the brain's performance.

Let's begin with the low energy. What causes this?

There are several thingsto consider, but foremost is the decline in mitochondria. As we've previously discussed mitochondria are tiny fuel-producing cells that reside throughout your cells. They are responsible for taking glucose and transform it into ATP or Adenosine Triphosphate, the 'energy money of life'.

They're found all over the body, and this includes the brain, where they reside within the brain cells. If you've ever been exhausted or in a hurry to finish a task due to the fact that it demands keeping figures in the working memory the 'brain' is not working as well.

It's what makes it difficult to find the motivation to take on any thing at all. Yet another night with the same television it's then...

If you looked at cells from a child under a microscope and then compare them to those of an older man, you'd find that middle-aged men had significantly less mitochondria. Scientists are now convinced that this could be one of the main differences in levels of energy of youngsters versus adults.

In reality, this is also one the main things that many nootropics are focusing on. Ingredients that range from l-carnitine PQQ, Lutein and even creatine to bitter orange function at least in part this way.

Another factor that can affect the brain's energy levels as we grow older is the flow of blood. Just like every other area that you have, your mind requires an ongoing supply of blood in order to supply oxygen and nutrients to ensure functioning at a high level. However, as your breathlessness after reaching the top step will prove, our blood flow is reduced when we get older.

Vasodilators are where they come in. The extracts of garlic vinpocetine, ginkgo biloba and vinpocetine all boost energy through the expansion of blood vessels. It can also be beneficial to those suffering from hypertension! They allow more oxygen, blood and nutrients to flow towards the brain, allowing you feel more alert and alert. As previously mentioned, you could also benefits from B12 and iron that help the body produce greater red blood cell. This is a simple process usually enough to increase the quantity in oxygen as well as nutrients that make their way from in the human body and to brain, and further boost you energy levels.

Learning and Mood

As we age and get older, we usually make less crucial neurochemicals, whether that's serotonin or the dopamine. Dopamine is among the neurotransmitters connected with attention, and also has a correlation with memory (the more concentrated you are and the better your concentration, the more likely you'll be to recall something - usually the things you've forgotten were things you didn't listen to in the first place). ...).

Dopamine also has a correlation with BDNF also. Bran Derived Neurotrophic factor. Along with the nerve growth factor, BDNF is one of the major factors in neuroplasticity. As we get older, the rate

33

of brains' ability to adapt and grow alters, which leads to a decrease in the capacity to acquire new abilities and concepts as well as a decrease in enthusiasm for learning.

You know what you can eat to boost your dopamine levels, improve your concentration and improve your learning? Good old caffeine! Perhaps, it is not a coincidence the consumption of caffeine is linked to a lower chance of developing Alzheimer's disease. Dopamine also affects your mood, and so are other neurochemicals that diminish as we age , like serotonin, also known as the "happiness hormone".. A lot of these neurochemicals are derived of amino acids that are simple (the proteins' building blocks) like tryptophan , l-tyrosine and tryptophan. Consume more eggs (which are also loaded with the brain-boosting Choline) Your brain is likely to become more robust and you'll feel less stressed.

Other nootropics are able to boost brain plasticity , and there are many intriguing studies that have proven that we may one day be able restore our brains to levels similar to those of infants that are plastic (one study suggested it could be possible to instruct participants to the art of pitch using certain nootropics that are not yet commercially available).

This will not only assist us learn new abilities - and teach an elderly dog new techniques, but also help us avoid from falling into oldand slow mental habits. One of the major challenges here is the way we think as we age. As we get older, we learn more (we develop more 'crystalized intelligence') which results in an easing of the need to continue studying. Additionally, years of practicing the same thinking patterns (and their neural pathways) can mean that certain thoughts and concepts are deeply embedded while others are cut off from the brain, and let to wilt and shrink. Utilize it or let it go.

This is the reason it's crucial to keep your brain well-nourished with the proper ingredients and nutrients even further into life. And to aid in that growth with the correct nutrient routine or supplements.

How do you go about doing this? The best solution is to eat a healthy and high-protein diet. This will help in stimulating the production of appropriate neurochemicals. This can aid in gaining greater mental clarity and energy and improve your mood.

Additionally, the right nutrition will also protect your brain from some of damage it could be exposed to over the course of time. The brain can be damaged by free radicals like any other cell within your body. They are molecules that react with the exterior of cell walls, causing damage , and possibly even impact on the brain's nucleus. Vitamin C and antioxidants can stop this type of damage.

In addition the omega 3 fatty acid which is the oil that fish consume can aid in improving the communication between cells through enhancing the permeability of cell membranes. It has also been proven to prevent the onset the decline in cognitive function caused by age in research.

If you're beginning to feel that your grey matter is beginning to slowing down, try eating more vegetables and fruits in addition to more salads, oilsy fish and meats. It's enough to bring about a significant impact, but if you're still not seeing results or are struggling to eat healthy and stay fit, you should consider making an'stack' of nootropics' for yourself. Be sure to include the following items:

Vitamin C (precursor for serotonin and also an antioxidant)

Garlic (a natural vasodilator)

Creatine (boosts the energy of cells)

CoQ10 or resveratrol (boosts cell energy)

Vitamin B6 and Vitamin B12 (for greater energy and better

5HT and L-Tyrosine (a form of tryptophan, Any amino acid supplement can be effective)

Iron, Magnesium Zinc, Vitamin D (these are also able to aid in testosterone production in males)

Lutein (this can also assist in achieving vision)

Omega 3 Fatty Acid (improves the cell membrane permeability)

Guarana (a slow-releasing type of caffeine)

Of course, you must avoid all items that could harm the brain and cause the neurochemical imbalances/trigger degeneration.

One of the most serious cause of this is alcohol, which is consumed frequently can cause a distinct kind of cognitive decline known as "Korsakov's syndrome".

Growing your interest, learning and Memory Through the Right Lifestyle

Do you know something that's more important than all this?

Engaging your brain on regularly.

It's also a matter of using it or losing it. One reason why we observe a lot of the degeneration that we experience in our brains is because we don't learn anything new and cease to expose our minds to new experiences. This is a terrible mistake.

We've touched on BDNF and the brain's plasticity. However, knowing the mechanism behind this process is the key to revealing how important it is to continue studying.

In essence, when you engage your brain, you trigger certain neurons in your brain to "fire" (called the action potential). If two neurons are firing simultaneously it creates a connection and the more often two neurons fire at the same time and the more powerful that connection grows. That's the way we acquire knowledge, and it's how memories are created The more times we repeat tasks and the easier it is to predict that each action or signal will trigger the next. This is made clear when we believe something is crucial and pay the task our complete attention this causes an increase in dopamine as well as other neurotransmitters that stimulate the brain. This triggers releases of BDNF to increase synaptic plasticity.

In the meantime, if the connection isn't being used Pruning can take place and the connection is gradually degraded.

The more you study and make connections and connections, the more BDNF and dopamine that your brain produces. However, when you stop taking in new information and you lose the capacity to master the new concepts. In the meantime you repeat the same actions and the same thoughts repeatedly, will make it extremely difficult to your mind diverge from these established paths.

This is the reason it's normal to see people who are older being extremely opinionated and established in their way. They've lost the ability make new connections, but their current relationships are fixed in stone.

Consider how this is related to changes in our life. When we're younger the world is constantly changing and we're always learning (the brain is a lover of novelty!). This continues even in university, and will continue as we enter our careers.

Then we are entangled in an established career path and begin to do the same routines every day. These tasks are no longer challenging and we're merely doing the same thing over and over. Dopamine production decreases and brain plasticity declines. At this point we also cease to be active.

When we get older then we cease to be active in any way and have a great time doing nothing. Our bodies aren't working or our brains, and pruning takes place faster than the formation of new connections. We become forgetful, and find it difficult to stay engaged or learn new things.

The most important thing is keeping your mind working. The majority of blogs and articles that you read on the internet will suggest activities like reading and chess for this purpose, however what's most important is to continue to learn new things. The brain loves novelty, and the more you give it the better chance it'll keep growing and learning, as well as adapting.

The best way to do this is to play computer games. The reason behind this is that each PC game needs a unique level of motor skills (owing to the different controls) and provides unique experiences, and new challenges and puzzles. Social games online are more enjoyable.

Chapter 5: Master the Art of Self-Love and Take on Depression

Nicole is a sweet heart. She's among the most caring and most remarkable people you'll meet. However, she's generous to the point of being a problem. She's a"people-pleaser. She puts the needs of others above her own. She makes excuses all the time. Sometimes she gets the impression that everyone is walking over her. She's exhausted and yet she's unable to tell anyone "no."

Then she developed clinical depression. She was unable to leave from her home. She stayed in bed in tears and thinking about negative thoughts about herself and her situation. She would eat chips and had soda throughout the day. She lost her youthful look. She looks as if she's aged 45, despite being just 28. Her pores grew bigger. Her skin started to loosen as she noticed some wrinkles on her face.

Then, Nicole finally got tired of crying and moping. Nicole made the decision to be a lover and made herself the top priority. She chose to view herself as a valuable and worthy human being. She began taking charge of her physical and health appearance. She started investing in bath and perfumes. She began to exercise at the gym and consume healthy food. She began saying "no" to any requests that could compromise her health and/or her health.

After a couple of months, she shed the extra weight. She started to appear more attractive and vibrant. Her glow was something she couldn't explain. She was more relaxed and happier. Additionally, she started to attract positive circumstances. And she looked younger and more youthful.

Whitney Houston once sang, "Learning to love yourself is the most important loving thing you can do." According to the lyrics, out, love is the most powerful emotion that is essential to beat depression. It's also the path towards eternal youthfulness.

You'll age faster If you're not confident and constantly look at other people. To lead a fulfilling life, it is essential to completely accept yourself -- imperfections and everything else. It's important to learn to accept and appreciate yourself for who you are. Here's how to accomplish this:

Recognize your strengths and talents.

If you're constantly worrying about your flaws then you'll soon feel depressed, and soon you'll be noticing wrinkles in your appearance. Therefore, take a seat and list all of your strengths. It could be something like "I am gentle," "I am good with children," "I am a superb dancer" as well as "I am a great coder."

Write down all your accomplishments and all the issues you've overcome, as well as the challenges you've overcame. This exercise will help you realize how great you truly are.

Make time to be aware of your appearance.

Every day, take a examine yourself in the mirror and take a moment to be awed by yourself and your appearance. What do you love about your appearance in general? Do you love your hair? Do you have gorgeous eyes with almonds? Do you have gorgeous skin? Keep your eyes on the good and not the negative. However, you must accept your physical limitations. So what happens if you're carrying an extra pound or big eyes? Being able to shed a bit of belly fat is a sign that you're blessed as you have enough money to buy tasty food. For the record, eyes that are wide are stunning.

Release your regrets.

Are you unhappy? Do you often get angry? Do you frequently attack anyone, including your beloved ones? Do you engage in unhealthy habits like eating out, smoking and drinking a lot? If you've answered "yes" on these concerns, then you're likely to be having regrets about your life.

Remorseful living could take away your joy. It can rob you of your peace and joy, and result in a few lines to appear across your forehead.

Be positive about yourself.

In order to boost your self-esteem, and to achieve lasting happiness, you must shut down those who criticize you and let out that inner fan. You have to become your most fervent admirer and motivater. To achieve this, you must daily affirm yourself with positive words.

Positive affirmations make you more hopeful, optimistic and confident. As with the thoughts you think of, words affect your reality. If you're looking to be younger, be aware of the words you choose to describe yourself.

The affirmations below boost confidence in yourself, and may remove years off your appearance.

I'm fine just the way I am.

I am young at heart.

Every single part of my body vibrates with joy and eternal youthfulness.

I am a young person with a lot of enthusiasm.

I am brimming with energy.

I am happy with myself. I'm comfortable with who I am. I'm happy with myself.

I have a childlike enthusiasm and exuberance.

I am thrilled by all the happenings in my life.

I embrace my mistakes.

I accept my own forgiveness for the many mistakes I've made in the past.

I do not dwell on the past. I prefer to move forward.

I am capable and competent. I can be a blessing to this world.

It's not too late for me to become the person I would like to be.

I deserve to be happy and successful.

I'm proud of myself.

Ich am the personal motivator and cheerleader.

I let go of my self-doubt.

I am able to transform my life.

I prefer happiness.

I am confident in myself.

Everything I need to have the greatest success.

I am in a position to design the kind of life I would like to live.

I take care of me with respect, and with kindness.

I appreciate myself.

I am getting ever more confident and confident each day.

I am a wonderful person.

I am currently in the process of creating positive habits for my life.

I am a problem-solver.

It is not necessary to repeat all of these affirmations. You only need to use the ones that are relevant to you.

Take a break.

Don't get too harsh on yourself. Have a break whenever you have to. Plan a trip to a holiday. Plan a trip for a weekend to another city if you're required to. But most importantly, don't be ashamed to relax! After all the hard work your body deserves it.

Make sure you take care for your health.

You are a valued human being. Therefore, you must be treated as such. You should be aware of your well-being. Stay away from fast food and sugary food items whenever you are able to. Take a big amount of fruit and vegetables.

Add enjoyable activities to your routine.

If you're feeling depressed, you're tempted to be at home. You stop engaging in the things you used to love. You want to lay in your bed and play Netflix throughout the day.

In order to beat depression, you should add enjoyable activities to your daily routine. It is important to make yourself do things that you love. It doesn't require an enormous amount or go to the extraordinary. Here's a list with a few enjoyable activities you can add into your routine

Take a date with your loved one.

Go to a movie that makes you feel good.

Find an inspirational quote.

Enjoy a long soak in the bubble bath.

Bake cookies to delight your loved ones.

Visit a museum for free and an art museum.

Invite your friends to a barbecue, and invite your most beloved acquaintances.

Help someone who is in need. This will give you the feeling of a "helper's exhilaration."

Try something new, such as painting or yoga.

Do something that you're exceptionally good at.

If you're in need of a confidence boost, try something you're extremely skilled at. You can cook or dance, sing or code, or even write. Perform any task you are confident you can complete efficiently. This boosts your confidence in yourself and creates a mix of positive hormones within your brain.

Limit your social media time.

Social media is fantastic as it lets you connect to your loved ones and friends however, it can also trigger jealousy. If you see photos of your pals' luxurious automobiles, massive houses, and extravagant vacations, it's hard from feeling bad about yourself.

Be aware that people only share only a tiny portion of their lives through social networks. Psychologists suggest that people tend to share positive aspects that they are happy with on their social networks. But there's more. Therefore, be patient and try to be thankful for the accomplishments of other people.

Set boundaries.

There will be wrinkles on your face if you continue answering "yes" in response to demands that don't align with your objectives, goals, dreams and beliefs. It is important to establish boundaries. It is important to know how to be able to say "no." It is important to need to confront those who are in constant disdain and unkind to you.

Do not try to hide your emotions.

It's perfectly normal to be annoyed and even frustrated at times. All emotions are beautiful. Don't try to hide your emotions. Celebrate and embrace these feelings.

Be around positive and inspirational people.

You'll age quickly when you're around negative and toxic people. You must surround your self with people who are optimistic about you -- people who encourage you and encourage you to believe you can accomplish incredible things.

Give yourself love and respect.

The golden rule is, "Do unto others what you would like other people to do to you." If you wish to live an enjoyable life it is essential to take care of yourself as you want others are going to treat you. You must be able to be self-loving and respectful when you want others to be able to appreciate and love you.

Self-love doesn't just increase your happiness but can also help you grow older. Therefore, you must be sure to take care of you and your requirements.

Chapter 6: Add The Meaning to Your Life: Affiliating Your Life's Purpose

"The goal of life is to discover what you are good at. Your job is to enhance it. The purpose of living is to give your gift to someone else." David Viscott. David Viscott

The purpose of living is ..... very well... it's a mystery to me. don't know... it's for everybody. For me, the most important thing in my life is to help humanity to my best abilities by enjoying and appreciating every moment currently, in the moment it is happening. I am extremely passionate about helping others improve their health and enjoyment of life. That's what I am focused on. It's possible for you to be different. Every person has different goals out of their lives. While I'm unable to say what your personal meaning in life however, I can say that I am certain that every person has a passion for something and nearly everybody has the capacity to turn that passion into an offering to themselves and to the world, if they choose to. I am also aware that when someone has a desire and desires to do something with their heart and mind the fire in their souls in a state of blaze. Even ordinary individuals and women have the ability to climb mountains and do extraordinary things.

The connection between your mind and the desire for living, as well as your ability to live has been extensively documented. This is what the scientific community refers to as "the Nocebo Effect." "Nocebo," is a modified version of"placebo" or "placebo," with it's Latin root reinterpreted to translate to "I will cause harm." It is the Nocebo effect is described as the physical and psychosomatic injury to someone in a study that believes that something benign (like sugar pills) could cause harm to them. Like how the placebo effect is an effective healing agent it is associated with severe rises in liver enzyme levels in severe blood pressure, heart rate drops, hyperventilation asthma, depression and even depression and other symptoms. Scientists believe that the combination rapid breathing and intense anxiety triggers an ensuing chain reaction within the hypothalamus and pituitary as well as the adrenal glands. These are the areas of the body that are able to deal with physical threats from the outside (think the "fight or flight" reaction taken to extreme). In the event that the terror is intense enough, it is believed that the combination of hormones could result in organ damage, and, in certain extreme cases even death. There are numerous documented cases of people who believed they were dead, whether because they believed that their lives was not worth living or they were told, or were convinced that they would be dead within a certain period of time. Certain of the cases I've read are truly terrifying however, to be honest there was no evidence that any of the incidents I've read about was conducted in a controlled environment in the recent past. There are, for obvious reasons, several ethical concerns surrounding these kinds of scientific research in the present. In any case the nocebo effect is extremely real and I'm not planning to personally test the strength of its effects up to their limits.

Happily... It's been a good thing! It's the same with the opposite. If someone is determined to live, in every cell of their body, and when they can find and bring the meaning of their lives and a goal they're determined to achieve it is possible to reverse the clock and put the grim reaper in a safe place. There are numerous instances of people who've overcome cancer and disease, despite unbelievable odds, and lived an additional 10, 20, 30or more years, to the awe of their doctors. There are countless stories of people being pushed to live because of their goals or dreams which they were obsessed with finishing. There are many great examples of this in the Napoleon Hill classic Think and Grow Rich. There are many inspirational stories that span from Jack

Lalane to Louis Zamperini (both his escape from the raft as well as his escape in the Japanese interment camps). The stories range from Mike Tyson keeping Cus D'Amato alive to the tale of Philippides passing away after he accomplished his task to run from Marathon in Greece to Athens to bring the news of triumph over the Persians. If you're looking for additional examples, look up Viktor Frankl's book Man's Search for Meaning. In the book, he discusses in great detail how only people who made it through in the Nazi internement camps are people who could come up with a reason to exist even in the most difficult of circumstances. The book also highlights how lucky the majority of us are living today in our lives. But , again, only should we decide to take the time to appreciate the goodness around us each day.

What does all this relate to our goals for a healthy age? I am of the firm belief that when you discover an objective for your life, something you'd love to do, and completely with your whole heart, and soul to attain, you will be blessed with more energy and vitality, which you can utilize to boost both the efficiency and duration of your life. The next step is to decide .... what are you looking to accomplish do in your life?

Chapter 7: Kiss All Your Stress Away

Stress is an integral part of modern life. A little bit of stress can be beneficial as it can motivate you to improve your performance. It pushes you to be more efficient in your job.

But constant exposure to stress could result in a variety of health issues. Stress can lead to anxiety and depression. It could also cause numerous health problems, including chest pain, fatigue, sleep issues, headaches diabetes, heart issues. Also, it makes people age faster.

In order to keep your attractive appearance, you'll need to put aside your worries. Here is a list of ways to achieve that.

Do some meditation.

Meditation is among the most effective techniques for managing stress. It is a way to relax every cell of your body. It eases anxiety and boosts self-confidence. Studies have shown that it also reduces ageing.

To minimize lines on the face, lie in a comfortable posture. You can do this by sitting on a chair or cushion. Shut your eyes. breathe deeply. Take a deep breath and let out tension. Get rid of all worry and worries. Concentrate upon your breathing. Focus on the present moment. If an unfocused thought comes into your mind, simply let it go. it and return your attention to your breathing.

When you take a deep breath and exhale, declare, "I am at peace with myself." When you exhale, repeat, "I am getting younger every daily." Repetition this 20 times at least. After you're done, pray a prayer of acceptance, peace, and gratitude. After that, you can open your eyes.

Avoid caffeine.

A majority of people require a cup of coffee in the morning to boost their energy during the entire day. However, drinking too much coffee could result in depression and anxiety. Also, it increases your cortisol levels, which can make you feel anxious and stressed. So, try to stay away from the caffeine as much as you can.

Music is a great way to relax.

Music can soothe your soul. It's powerful enough to alter your mood and help you feel more relaxed. It takes away all worries and can also ease physical discomfort. If you're anxious take your headphones off and enjoy your favourite tunes.

Take a look at a hilarious video.

The saying goes laughter is the most effective medicine. It's also a natural antidepressant too. It helps to relieve all of stress and makes you look younger and more joyful. If you're feeling like you're overloaded with stress and responsibilities you can take a break and enjoy a hilarious cat or dog footage on YouTube.

Drink green tea.

This amazing coffee originates from Asia is a rich source of L-theanine that is a relaxing and soothing agent for your body.

It helps reduce the effects of anxiety and stress. Additionally, it has potent antioxidants that can help reduce the signs of the process of aging.

Take advantage of challenges as an opportunity.

The Chinese language, the word "challenge" is synonymous with chance. In fact, every difficulty (or problem) presents an opportunity to improve and grow stronger.

Visualize.

Visualization is an effective mental exercise that relaxes all parts that is your body. It relieves stress, and helps you be happy.

If you're stressed out take a deep breath and focus on the sounds surrounding you. Imagine sitting on a beach. The beach is a pleasant place to be. white sand that is on your back. It is possible to hear the waves' sound. Birds fly across the sky. You're relaxed. You're worry-free. You're content.

You can hold this image for as long as you are able to.

Then, take deep breaths and let your body ease into relaxation. Let go of all tension and stress from your body. Once you're fully relaxed, you can open your eyes.

Live in the moment.

Don't spend your time thinking about the past or fretting over the next year. It's impossible to change the past. The thought of thinking over the next few years is not a good idea. Just do your best todayso that you can have a better happy, more relaxed, and less stressful future.

Do some playtime and play with your dog.

Pets playing with you can provide you with genuine joy. It also can help relieve anxiety. If you've were unhappy at work, take some moments with your fluffy pet.

Massage your body.

Massages can boost the flow of blood. It helps you feel calm and rejuvenated while at the same time. Each stroke will wash your stress and tension away.

Massages can help improve the sleep quality, and aids in healing injuries too.

Stress can wreck havoc on your life. It could even cause death and cause you to look older. If you're looking to take years off your body and face it is essential to be able to manage stress levels and live a healthier life.

Chapter 8: The Habits that will improve your mood and Look

Training regularly

In reality among the most crucial ways we can improve our appearance and the way we appear when we're getting older is to work out. A recent study done by the American College of Sports Medicine discovered that exercise is among the most effective methods to increase mobility as we get older. When I talk about "exercise" isn't have to refer to a vigorous weightlifting session or even a half marathon. Simple activities like a quick 15-minute stroll or yoga class can make a huge difference. Through improving mobility, it is not just that we appear younger, but we'll also improve many aspects of our lives which test the body's capabilities. Things like climbing an uphill climb or sitting down to take out newspapers are all things that could be difficult for certain people, but as long as remain fit, these won't ever become a problem over time.

Sleeping enough

If you're in most American adults, it's probable that you don't get enough sleep each night to fully recover from an extended day. It's true, it's possible that your sleeping habits could cause you to gain weight. Instead of focusing on having an adequate night's rest, we are focused on getting our energy by drinking a cup of tea or sweet treats that ultimately results in weight growth. It also means that if your tired, you'll likely not have the time to cook healthy meals which is why you'll choose an eat-in restaurant at work and you'll end up eating a million calories. This is an unending cycle that results in lower levels of activity and a higher intake of calories. It is normal for our brains to the lack of sleep by searching to comfort food. What is the immediate consequence of this? Sure, you'll be able to be awake but what will it cost you? Fat, unwelcome, moodiness fatigue, irritability, tiredness and many other signs.

It's no fact that our bodies repair their own bodies when we sleep. In allowing our bodies enter a deep sleep state, we give our bodies the chance to heal from the stress that we endure throughout the day. As we rest in a deep sleep, our cells in our skin to create collagen, the fibrous tissue of our bodies that is an essential ingredient in a firm, youthful-looking skin. The amount of sleep adults should have can vary between 7.5 to 8 hours of continuous rest. Keep in mind that sleep debt is similar to credit card debt. If you don't stop accumulating debt, you'll eventually be bankrupt.

In order to have the best night's sleep, you must create the ideal environment that encourages healthy sleeping. First suggestions I offer is removing the television in your room You must unwind yourself before going to bed. And by watching TV before going to mattress, we allow our brains be stimulated until they fall asleep. Eliminate your laptop as well as the Smartphone too. It is possible to do a bit of light reading in an evening light but that's all. Avoid eating any large meals or drinks with caffeine before going to going to bed, as this can make your digestive system be overworked and could influence your sleep.

Stop smoking cigarettes

Smoking cigarettes is without doubt one of the most harmful ways to live your life particularly in the case of trying to keep young. Smoking cigarettes has been proven to speed up the process of aging. the cells undergo and has been proven to accelerate the process of aging in those younger than 20. Cigarettes are packed with more than 5000 ingredients, which when inhaled can result in harmful compounds that can alter your skin's composition and also your fingers, teeth the mouth, lungs eyes and the your immune system. Smoking also impacts the skin of our face by decreasing the quantity of blood that the skin receives which could eventually result in skin wrinkles and spots.

Quitting smoking can be among the most difficult things you can do However, there are many alternatives available to those who are looking to stop. If staying healthy is among your goals, then quitting smoking cigarettes will provide you with almost instant outcomes and I am sure you'll feel more relaxed and healthier in no time.

Make sure you are protected from the sun

You're probably aware of the dangers of UV radiation on your skin. But a new study by Scientists in Nambour, Australia concluded through microtopography that people who don't wear sunscreen or sunglasses show the damage to the skin's deeper layers collagen, elastic fibers, as well as collagen. The patients wearing sunscreen had as much as 24 percent less skin damage.

When we expose our skin to the continuous UV radiation from the sun, we're in danger of damaging our skin prematurely which is causing a slowdown in the process of regeneration that occurs in the cells of our skin. Additionally, continuous UV radiation has been found to be associated with a variety of serious conditions like skin cancer, Melanoma, premature ageing and other skin-related damage. This isn't just restricted to the face. The skin on our forearms the neck, shoulders, and hands are susceptible to damage from long-term exposure UV radiation.

Exposure to sun for long periods of time eventually causes the skin on our bodies to get thicker wrinkled and streaked. Since the damage is usually incurred slowly, many people don't realize the damage until it's already too to late. Always ensure that you wear sunscreen if you plan to be exposed to the sun's rays and be sure to wear UV-rated glasses since the skin around the eyes is very susceptible to radiation.

Avoid stress

Stressful and general anxiety can have a tremendously taxing impact upon your body. Stress-related fatigue and excessive stress can affect the DNA within skin cells, causing them to shrink the cell telomeres. This causes cells to break down or even to die. And not just that, even the mere thought of stress can increase the risk of developing disorders due to aging by making the brain work in overdrive. Recent research has shown that stress levels higher could cause the human brain to go toward aging-related signs.

It is vital that we understand how to manage anxiety and stress situations by relaxing ourselves and adapting to the situation. Experts advise us to take time for periods of deep relaxation and meditation. Finding the stress-causing factors within your life could contribute to improving your overall mental well-being. Examine your behavior and attitude and take the responsibility of your behavior. If stress becomes too much, it may be beneficial to seek professional assistance.

If nothing else works you can think about having a day off. it can be very beneficial in managing stress, but don't stay in bed worrying about how miserable tomorrow will be. Instead, plan your day in advance Make sure you plan your day around eating a nutritious filling meal and engaging in some exercise, such as a short exercise, such as cycling or swimming. You could even take your dog on a stroll! The goal is to get away from the countless things we are faced every day. Through "resetting" the minds and bodies, we will be able to effortlessly overcome the effect of stress.

Chapter 9: Change Your Habits

If you've realized that anti-aging is a fact and you must be very serious about it, let's take a look at the point.You'll learn what you must do to stop the process of aging that the passage of time and your lack of interest may have already begun. There's some positive and some negative information here.The positive side is the fact that all you have to take to slow the aging process is as easy as it is. The guidelines are simple as well as logical and simple to remember. Another benefit is that you do not have to spend a lot of money on the quest to get older. In reality, the expensive remedies that shout at you in commercials are made up of much less expensive ingredients that you definitely can pay for. The fanciful medicines and devices which claim to will help you lose weight or appear younger in only a couple of weeks are all scams. Don't fall for it. The good news is that there aren't any shortcuts to this path. You must take every step you can, at your natural pace. It is vital to not expect to see results in a short time. This is the toughest part. You must be perseverant and committed.

Certain decisions, such as whether you'll hit fitness today, or not aren't easy to make repeatedly, each day. It's imperative that you establish some new habits because only work that lasts for a long time can count. The things you do to improve your health now is important, also, but only as part of the bigger picture of your efforts to fight aging. There are some rules you should adhere to regardless of the situation.

Rule One is to eat Healthy Food

You don't have to worry about it; there's no need to worry about the calories you consume. However there are many things you know well aren't healthy, such as French fries, white bread, or anything else which is loaded with sugar but you still consume them. Stop eating them all together. They cause confusion for your body and cause a mess in your metabolism. The negative effects of eating junk food are weight gain as well as diabetes, heart attack and many more. It's not a good method of staying youthful. Be aware that anti-aging refers to avoiding everything that causes the process of aging. It's that easy. On the other hand of the equation, there are amazing nutritious, extremely valuable nutrients like olive oil, green vegetables or fish, that you are aware of the need to be eating regularly, yet do not. Now is the time to begin eating them. You'll find out more about these dishes and the best way to cook the same at Chapter 4, careful what you eat.

Rule No. 2: Rest at the end of the night

Are you aware of what your body is doing in the event that it does not perform any action? What does your body do when you rest? It regenerates. It is able to focus on different things during the day, as you are focused on your daily problems. Your entire capacity is engaged with different tasks while you're awake. A different set of metabolic processes take place after you fall asleep. If you are sleeping more and you allow for your body and mind recuperate.

Our bodies are wired to become exhausted at the moment the Sun gets dark. Nature has controlled everything beautifully however, we live in a age filled with artificial lights and a staggering number of illnesses that are caused by sleep absence. The balance between activities and sleep is vital to preventing aging. You must develop a healthy pattern of sleep immediately.

Rule #3 3: Workout Everyday

It is essential to exercise to prevent aging. Regular physical activity is a signal that signals the primitive brain structures that the world is good and we should be able to build up our strength. In contrast being sedentary, it informs our brain that a catastrophe is coming, and that we must build up the most fat we can to endure it. Learn more about the effects of exercise, and the reasons why it's so crucial in preventing aging, and receive practical suggestions on how to train in order to be functionally younger In Chapter 4, Movement Is Life.

Rule number four Rule Number Four: Drink enough water

We all know that water comprises more than 50% of our bodies (the percentage varies based on our age, sexuality health, physical health). Furthermore, as you'll learn in the subsequent sections, the"conditiosine qua non"of anti-aging and the primary goal is a healthy circulation. Aerobic exercise improves our circulation, but a regular drinking of water is vital to allow our bloodstream to function effectively. It's clear that the majority of our blood is made up of water and we should not put yourself in danger of becoming dehydrated. This is the reason you should to drink at minimum 2 or 3 liters water per every day. Begin your day with the glass of water. take a drink throughout the day, and force yourself to drink when you need to, and remember to carry an empty bottle when you run or go to the gym.

Rule Number Five: Good Hygiene Habits

Remember the first rule you were taught when you were a child. Hygiene can help you keep your health in check and avoid diseases. A healthy lifestyle is crucial to being younger and looking better. If you're looking for to see a more evident connection between good hygiene practices and anti-aging, think of two identical twins. One has white teeth, while the other shows an disgusting yellow stains whenever they smile. Whatever their age or general appearance How do you feel about? Which one is more attractive? Which one is younger?

Rule Six: Take Be Careful About Your Skin

Your skin is one of the most striking and surprising sign for your age. However it's also an unfortunate fact that it is one of the most difficult to combat the signs of aging. It is essential to acknowledge that you cannot stop a certain amount of skin deterioration. But you can reduce the ageing process on your skin (and reduce the chance of skin cancer in your way) by limiting your exposure to the Sun by wearing sunscreen regularly and avoiding alcohol (dehydration causes your skin to look terrible, even before it starts to affect other areas in the body). Be aware that everything you eat and drink has an impact on your skin. Additionally all the things you do to improve your overall health and fitness affects your skin. It is also possible to use some of the solutions listed in Chapter 6 Healthy Foods and remedies

Rule Number Seven: Avoid Alcohol

While alcohol-related advocates would love to highlight that drinking alcohol has benefits, such as it boosts circulation for instance, it can have a myriad of negative effects, ranging from dehydration to serious brain damage in addition to the dangers of alcoholism.

The first seven rules are all about taking control of your body. But, they won't aid your health if you neglect the effects that stress can have on your body and on the other hand the healing qualities of your mental well-being.

Rule Number Eight: Reduce Stress

While some stress may stimulate growth, chronic stress can cause death. The reality is that many people are living constantly under stress. They're under constant stress at work as well as at home. It is crucial to realize that constant stress transmits the same type of signals to the basic structures of your brain , as do people who live in a sedentary environment and lack of exercise sleeping insufficiently, and a poor diet. Furthermore, these risky issues tend to be combined. A lot of people suffer from each. Each of them will hinder the effects of your efforts to fight aging. The only way to make all of it and everything else function is to get out of your magic ring and modify your work (if feasible) or make it more bearable by improving your relationships with your coworkers. The average person spends at least 8 hours each day working and how you use those hours can have a significant impact on the overall quality of life. It's even more crucial what you do with the remainder of the day. Harmony at home is essential to your wellbeing, and rule number 9:

Rule Number Nine Rule Number Nine: Establish Relevant Relationships

Because you cannot accomplish it all by yourself. Create a genuine partner. Be supportive instead of assigning blame. Makea basis to grow together. If you don't have a partner, keep this in mind when you search for one. A good friend can be very beneficial. You need the motivation to grow older. You require someone to share your life with as you are determined to remain younger. As we have previously discussed the process of aging requires constant effort, and certain aspects of it can be difficult. It is essential to adhere to a strict program of healthy eating and exercise. It can be difficult to maintain your commitment. Sometimes, you'll require someone else to push you. Sometimes, you'll be required to push another. In this way, your work is more meaningful and you're more likely to be successful.

Chapter 10: Supplements For Healthier Skin.

It's not every day that we are able to enjoy the right diet with all the nutrients we require. For example, when we're traveling we are able to feast on the food available in the area we're going. Because of this, it is possible that we require some minerals and vitamins to maintain our skin. Be aware that neglecting your skin for a short period of time will cause some effects that can be seen. We must ensure that we keep our skins to be in the best way possible. Another reason we may require these supplements could be due to the absence of a specific nutrients within our bodies. Certain nutrients and vitamins like vitamin C and Omega 3 fatty acids, are crucial that if there is a lack of them inside our systems, our skin is affected a lot. In such instances it is possible to use supplements for a period of time to reverse the damage caused prior to removing the nutrients out of our diets.

Let's examine some of the supplements that result in more youthful looking skin.

Vitamin C supplement

Vitamin C supplements can be a great help in reverse the effects of the aging process. It also slows down the process of aging. It's antioxidants are powerful that eliminate all free radicals that are present in the skin. This ultimately leads to the skin being more elastic and firmer. We don't seem enough vitamin C in our diets. That's why I propose you take a supplement of vitamin C to maintain youthful-looking skin. This is especially important for those who've noticed that their skin appears older than it actually is. This vitamin is required regularly throughout the 30th day of feeling and looking younger. When we've recognized the signs of aging and have achieved our goals we can then stop taking supplements and include it in our diet.

The sun is a sworn enemy to our skin. Although we all enjoy being in the sun to get a sun-kissed bodies or simply soak up being warm, the impact on the skin can be massive. The UV rays of the sun damage the skin's proteins, leaving wrinkles on our faces. Vitamin C is among the most potent nutrients that can combat this issue. It can aid in rejuvenating the skin. If your skin is damaged and has wrinkles that are caused by a bad diet or prolonged time outdoors, consider taking supplements of vitamin C.

Omega 3 fat acids supplements

The Omega-3 fatty acids constitute essential nutrient that is beneficial to our skin. This particular nutrient can be derived from diets that contain seafood and fish. But, it is still able to be used as an added supplement. Apart from the reasons we've mentioned for using these essential nutrients as supplements, those who frequently develop blackheads or whiteheads on their skin will significantly benefit from taking omega 3 fat acid supplement. These nutrients are utilized by the skin to repairs, elasticity, and moisturizing purpose.

Zinc supplement

Zinc is a vital ingredient in healthy skin. The majority of zinc deposits found within the body are formed within the skin. Zinc assists the skin by regulating the quantity of oil that is released and produced through the skin. A deficiency in this mineral can cause dry skin, rashes, and wound healing issues. Dandruff can also indicate an imbalance in zinc levels inside our organisms. If you suffer from any of these signs, an intake of zinc supplements is beneficial for your skin. Zinc plays a variety of other roles in the body , particularly improving your immune system. It is beneficial for skin because infections aren't doing anything good for the skin. If we're well-being on the interior, it shows in our appearance. shows it to the outside.

Silica supplement

Silica is an elemental trace mineral present in our skin and in other areas of our bodies. It's vital for healthy skin. As we age our bodies lose substantial quantities of silica. This is the reason for wrinkles as well as decreases in elasticity the skin. Silica isn't a very well-known mineral, and it is only recently that people have started to recognize its importance in the process of aging. The people who are aware of it were successful in preventing their skin looking younger very well.

Silica can be found in many food items like mangoes, beans, cucumbers as well as asparagus and leeks, as well as strawberries, celery, and the rhubarb. Younger adults and children can take a slices of these sources. However, people who are older are, even if they consume these food items they are unable to take it in at the rate required. That means that more silica is discarded in the body than it is absorbed through food. People who are older need supplements with silica to meet their body's needs. It will help them appear and appear younger than they are. This is a secret that actually works. Silica is not just good for the skin but also hair and nails, but most important bones.

Supplementing with supplements to address an absence of a specific nutritional element that is not present in your body or your diet is something dermatologists recommend for. If we are continuously deficient in these nutrients over a prolonged period of time, our skin may age quickly making any subsequent treatments less efficient.

Chapter 11: Food and Nutrition Organic

In this section you'll find some helpful strategies to help you keep and maintain your youthful look for a long period of time. These tricks and tips are easy to follow and when used together with the recipes described above the skin will appear gorgeous and flawless, even when you're in your fifties.

Buy and eat organic

Although often viewed as a diet that is a trend but it has been proven numerous times that organic foods are much better for your general physical and mental well-being, in comparison to other types of food available in the marketplace. Instead of consuming food products that were produced using harmful fertilizers and pesticides make sure you purchase and eat a healthy diet.

A lot of organic and non-organic food items taste similar. But remember that even if it is impossible to detect the chemical, it may create a range of health issues. These chemicals aren't washable off. They are damaging to hair, skin and overall health. Hence it is recommended to consume organic food as often as possible.

Drink Water

Most people are aware of how important it is to drink at 8 ounces of water every day. This will make you look healthy, fit and young. This technique is beneficial to keep your skin hydrated , too. Therefore, it is important to drink the most water you can. If you are not a fan of drinking water's taste or you don't drink plain water it is possible to make lemonade and drink it instead. A better alternative is to buy the infuser bottles. With an infuser bottle you can add flavor along with the nutrients from any vegetable or fruit into the water, making it more delicious and healthier.

If you are unable to remember to incorporate water into your daily diet or fail to drink a glass every now and then You can download apps for your smartphone that will help you remember to drink more water. The majority the apps available are available for free and track the amount of water you've consumed throughout the day and how much is required for a healthy and fit body.

Drinking enough water will help keep your skin free of blemishes and clean. It can also give your skin with an never before radiant glow. It's also important for keeping your hair silky and shiny.

Eat Blueberries

Blueberries are thought to be a an extremely well-known and potent 'Superfood due to their substantial amount of the antioxidant resveratrol. This antioxidant is a effective body chemical that's an effective immune booster. It's also believed to combat cancer. It can slow the aging process and also lower blood sugar levels also. Wine and chocolate are abundant sources of the chemical, however , they're not great for general health therefore they should only be consumed in small amounts such as there is a significant amount of resveratrol in a half bottle of red wine is easily found in large portions of blueberries.

Be aware of your body

While it is essential to see your physician regularly to check-up on your health It is equally important to know your body's needs and be aware of the smallest changes. Making sure you are taking care of your health and protecting your body is among the most effective methods to keep looking and feeling youthful. Be aware of your hair, nails and eye color in order to know your overall health. If you can, read health-related books that will help you recognize your health issues and signs. Keep in mind that healthy hair and skin are indicators of the health of your body.

Create your Diet and life more vibrant

Many dieticians recommend creating a plate that is as colorful as you can. This is not referring to the dish's color , but to the quantity and variety of food items are required to consume. Incorporating different kinds of fruits and vegetables into your meals will help fight off different diseases and disorders. They also aid in battling wrinkles, and will keep you healthy and fit for a longer period of time. Included nuts in your diet can help you fight the signs of getting older. Nuts are a great supply of fat acids as well as nutrients. These are able to boost longevity and improve overall health.

Avoid Toxins

As mentioned earlier the presence of chemicals and toxins is extremely harmful to your well-being and health, therefore, they must be avoided at all times. But, toxins aren't only found in food items, but are also present in the air itself. Thus, it's important to safeguard your hair and skin every time you leave. Make sure to wash your hair and face often to keep away harmful toxins.

Chapter 12: Value of Diet, Exercise, and Hydration

Exercise and anti-aging

Exercise can delay the onset of age-related illnesses like diabetes, hypertension as well as coronary heart diseases. Exercise aids the body in eliminating harmful nitrogenous substances through sweat. It also assists in eliminating free radicals which are at the root of the damage to cells. Exercise plays a significant function in controlling the body's energy.

Regular exercise can not only help us look better and look better, but it also has an enormous impact on how we view ourselves and enhance the self-image we have. When we exercise, our brain releases the well-known hormones of dopamine, dopamine, and serotonin. These chemicals are also known as the happy hormones. These hormones are the reason why we feel confident about our bodies after working out. It's only when you exercise regularly that the levels of these hormones increase within the body, and we end up feeling satisfied, not just after exercise and for a long time afterwards.

Diet and anti-aging

Our diet is the most important thing we consume and it is important to always live our lives by this statement. If we eat a balanced and healthy diet we can reduce the process of aging. A diet that is rich in vegetables and fruits, which contain natural antioxidants and can assist a good fight against aging. The reason is that antioxidants offer immense benefits for our bodies.

By eating a healthy diet it is possible to turn back the clock of time. Food that is healthy has less calories and more nutrients , which can aid in maintaining an ideal body weight. Foods that are rich in vitamins affects the whole body, and by eating a healthy eating habits, we can enhance our healthand it can be seen how our complexion looks. It is also possible to use these nutritious foods to create homemade face scrubs and masks. And afterward, we can see the effects more clearly.

A healthy diet must include plenty of fresh vegetables and fruits as they contain a high levels of various vitamins, including Vitamin C. Fish is also important to our diet because it is rich in omega-3 fatty acids which protect our skin from sun-induced damage. The body needs healthy proteins. We can are able to get protein from eggs, meat seafood, beans, and eggs. We should also substitute white bread for regular whole grain breads and cereals. Instead of white rice, we should utilize brown rice.

Hydration and anti-aging

Without water, there's no existence. Human bodies require sufficient fluids to maintain its regular processes running smoothly. Water has an effect on every organ in our body, however typically, we aren't aware that we're dehydrated. Researchers agree that when you feel thirsty, you are dehydrated. Therefore, it is essential to drink all day long The reason we feel thirsty is simply the body's way of warning us of dehydration. Many people nowadays prefer to drink sodas or other similar drinks that contain lots of sugar. They are not a substitute for plain water, however, since they dehydrate our organs more, rather than providing the water we require.

The effects of drinking enough water will be visible the skin of your face You will appear healthier and more refreshed , and your skin will be glowing with that particular glow. It's easy to spot someone who isn't drinking enough water just by watching their appearance. They look dehydrated and their skin is dry and tight. Due to this, sufferers are more prone to wrinkles. If you're suffering having dry, flaky skin take a look at drinking more water as cells benefit greater from drinking water than other products you can apply to your skin.

How many ounces of water should we consume each throughout the day?

A lot of doctors recommend drinking 8 glasses of water per day, which is approximately 2 liters of drinking water, but the amount we drink will depend on many variables and the same principle is not applicable to each person. How much water consume during a given day will depend on the level of physical exercise, on the climate that we are in, and on the weight we carry and weight, etc. It is recommended to pay attention to your body since the body is constantly giving us signals that we must not ignore. In all cases, the recommended 8 glasses of water be used as a reference for starting with, and then modify depending on your individual needs.

Chapter 13: Three Things You Can Implement Immediately To Make You Look and Feel Younger

In our modern age, people seem to be searching for ways to appear younger. Many people apply different cosmetics to stop wrinkles or dark spots showing up. There are numerous creams, moisturizers, and other cosmetics that are able to slow the wrinkles You can choose to use natural products and be more careful about the foods you consume instead.

1. Take a large amount of water.

60% of our body's mass is composed of water. Any imbalance in this area can lead to illnesses. Diabetes mellitus, hypertension, and renal dysfunctions all contribute to changes of the levels of fluid in the body. Consuming plenty of fluids does not just help to prevent the diseases which are prevalent in people over the age of 65 as well as preventing damage to cells.

Water has many roles to play within the body. It is an important transport channel for various nutrients. It aids in the elimination of by-products from cellular metabolism that can be harmful to our body. It is also required by cells to enable them to function properly. One consequence from a deficiency in fluid intake can be dehydration. This can cause a shift of fluids from intracellular to extracellular compartment, which causes cell shrinkage. If it is severe, dehydration could cause comatose and even death.

As an example, perhaps you are being dehydrated and the liver cells are affected. Liver cells are among the busiest cells of the body. They are responsible for a variety of functions that include detoxification, production of energy , and the transformation of toxic metabolites into less harmful ones. If the cells of the liver shrink or die because of dehydration, all of these functions will be diminished.

Detoxification is one of the processes which aids in slowing down the process of aging. It's a procedure which neutralizes the effects of waste within the body. When the cells of your liver fail to do their job in removing waste products Then more toxins build up within the body, causing additional harm to the tissues. This is the case when the body is not able to flush out these harmful metabolites because of the lack of water. When you're dehydrated circulation slows down and this results in a decrease of blood filtration through the kidneys.

2. Consume foods that are rich in antioxidants, vitamins and minerals.

One of the symptoms of aging are the appearance many ailments. One method to stop them is to consume healthy food items. Fruits and vegetables, whole grains and fish are some of the food items that are recommended to avoid the appearance of age-related illnesses however, they also help to slow down the process of aging.

The majority of products for skin today are claimed to be high in antioxidants. But what people aren't aware of is there's many foods which are in reality common food items which contain large amounts of antioxidants. Vitamin C, Vitamin E and Vitamin A are among some of the strongest antioxidants in the world. They slow the aging process by stabilizing free radicals generated by cell metabolism.

Vitamin C is present in a variety of citrus fruits, including guava, citrus fruits and lemons. The two most potent sources of this vitamin are pomegranate , and the kiwi. It is important to include them in your diet. In contrast vitamin E is often located in darker green vegetables such as spinach, kale mustard and broccoli. Vitamin A is believed to improve eyesight, is found in orange and yellow fruits as well as vegetables such as tomatoes, carrots and squash. These three vitamins help to stimulate the renewal of skin cells and help you look younger and healthier.

Another antioxidant present in a variety of vegetables and fruits is lycopene and resveratrol, which are both present in tomatoes. Both antioxidants can reduce the development of various forms of cancer as well as decrease the chance of developing cardiovascular illnesses, including coronary heart attack and artery disease. Resveratrol is also present in coffee, red wine and grapes. Research suggests that drinking a glass of red wine a day can prevent cardiovascular disease.

Maintaining blood pressure is an issue that is a big concern for those who age. As we age the tone of blood vessels increase, resulting in an increase in the pressure against which the heart pumps blood to. One of the primary reasons for an increase in blood pressure in older adults is the buildup of cholesterol within blood vessels. Therefore, it is suggested to eat foods that are high in fiber like whole grains, barley, wheat and Oats. A majority of vegetables and fruits are also high in fiber. The indigestible substance slows the aging process by reducing the amount of cholesterol present in blood. What does it do?

Fiber is a binding agent for bile, a substance produced by the liver to help emulsify fats within the diet and to facilitate its elimination. Bile, comprised of cholesterol is usually recycled and transferred to the gallbladder to store. In normal circumstances only 2 percent of the amount of bile that is produced by the liver is eliminated every day, meaning that the majority of it is sent back to circulation. However, with fiber there is a greater amount of bile that is excreted is increased, causing your liver's ability to create more bile. In order to produce Bile, the liver needs to mobilize and use the cholesterol reserves in the body. The cholesterol levels in the blood to drop and, eventually the blood pressure goes downas well.

The blood pressure can also be maintained through eating foods that are rich in omega-3 acids which are found most often in the flesh of fish. Fish such as salmon, tuna and mackerel are among the most popular and effective suppliers of omega-

3. It is a long-chain polyunsaturated fat that can be easily emulsified by the human body. Omega-3 fatty acid has been proven to lower the risks of hypertension, stroke as well as Alzheimer's disease.

The aging process can cause loss of bone mass that is mostly due to the decrease in levels of hormones including estrogen. To stop the reduction in bone density you must consume foods that are high of calcium as well as vitamin D. These are present in anchovies, milk and dairy productssuch as butter and cheese. It is crucial to read the labels of dairy products you purchase. They are generally filled with cholesterol. Make sure that the dairy products you purchase don't contain saturated or trans-fats because these kinds of fats are able to solidify in the blood vessels.

3. Stay clear of high fat, processed, and sugar-rich foods that are high in sugar, fat and processed.

These days, processed food items are becoming more popular and, as a result the risk of developing diabetes mellitus, hypertension and cancer has risen. Many processed foods are high in chemical compounds like nitrosamines, benzene , which have been proven to trigger various types of cancer. There is also sodium, which is a mineral that is linked to hypertension. It is one of the most important electrolytes in the body. However, high blood levels of sodium can draw water from an intracellular compartment into the intravascular space or the space within the vessels, leading to increased blood flow. This can lead to hypertension due to the greater workload on the heart.

Foods that are high in sugar, on the other hand, may trigger diabetes mellitus. The sugars found in food are broken down into glucose in the body, and transformed into metabolites for the creation of energy. The process of metabolism, as previously mentioned creates greater amounts of free radicals thereby creating damage to cells. A rise in glucose levels in blood can cause diabetes mellitus an illness that is defined by a blood sugar level higher than 110 mg/dl blood thickening and a decline the flow of blood. When blood flow is reduced is the flow of nutrients and oxygen to cells decreases and causes damages.

Fat-laden foods are high in cholesterol, and it has been reported to cause an rise of blood pressure. A buildup of cholesterol in blood and the accumulating of cholesterol within blood vessels' walls may trigger inflammation. Inflammatory cells known as macrophages and neutrophils release chemical compounds that degrade cholesterol deposits. Chemical reactions can create free radicals. However, instead of bringing benefits on the body, by eliminating cholesterol, the inflammation process actually created more harm.

Chapter 14: Brain Health

The body's control centre is made up of the brain and the nervous system. They control the body's movements, store thoughts and memories, analyses the body's senses, and assists to regulate the other bodily systems and organs. The brain transmits signals to the body through nerves which are pathways that connect through the entire body. For example, the spine is one such pathway of nerves that runs from your brain all the way into your middle back.

Aging causes changes in the nervous system and brain like atrophy, in which nerve cells get removed. The number of nerve cells decreases and the messages that are transmitted through the brain to the rest of the body could be sent in a less rapid manner. Additionally nerve cells begin degrade in the brain, releasing waste products that can cause neurological disorders including plaques and lipofuscin. The breakdown of nerve cells could affect the sensitivities, which decreases feelings and reflexes as well as the senses of smell, sight and taste. Memory, cognitive processing and thinking can also decrease as we age due to these changes to the brain and nervous system.

Anti-aging Brain and Nervous System Health 101: Essential Oils and Preventative Methods

Like the rest of our human body, brain requires an exercise program and healthy diet to prevent the effects of aging. Neurodegeneration is an inevitable consequence of aging. However, it can happen at a lower intensity and with a lesser rate if preventative strategies are consistently exercised.

To ensure the health of your nervous system and your brain, think about both mental and physical exercise. Exercise will supply adequate amounts of oxygen to your brain. This can reduce cell loss in the brain and mental exercises - such as solving word puzzles, studying and debating, taking part in ongoing intellectual discussions or debates. Keep your brain sharp as a needle.

There are "superfoods" which can improve brain function, and many are also beneficial for the health of your skin. This includes nuts and seeds avocados and fish (or other fish rich in omega-3s) whole-grains, blueberries tomatoes, broccoli and sage.

The antioxidant nature of essential oils can help you fight the effects of aging with regard to the nervous system and brain. Check out the following study released by Journal of Oleo Science, where the antioxidant benefits on the effects of Lemon essential oil in neurodegeneration were studied.

Study 4 - Antioxidant Properties

"This study sought to investigate the effects of essential oil from Lemon (Citrus limon) peels on acetylcholinesterase (AChE) and butyrylcholinesterase (BChE) activities in vitro... The suppression in AChE and BChE actions, the inhibition of pro-oxidant-induced lipid peroxidation and antioxidant activity could be potential mechanisms for the utilization of essential oils in the prevention and treatment of neurodegeneration caused by oxidative stress."

By testing Lemon essential oil against acetylcholinesterase and butyrylcholinesterase, both of which are enzymes which actively terminate neurotransmission, the study found that Lemon essential oil inhibits the damaging activity of these enzymes. This, along with the oil's antioxidant qualities, suggests it is possible that Lemon essential oil could have potential to aid in strengthening our body's own defense mechanisms against neurological disorders like Alzheimer's, ALS, Huntington's or Parkinson's.

Along with exercise and diet these essential oil regimens can help support the health of your brain and nervous system function. They can help you prime your brain to counteract the effects of aging.

Essential Oil Protocols

Brain Function

Description:

The following guidelines can help to improve brain performance as well as mental clarity.

Application:

* General health : dilute the essential oil according to (Grounding Blend Melissa and Frankincense are all suggested) and apply it topically to the brain stem as well as the soles of your feet.

Recommended oils:

Ylang Ylang, Sandalwood, Rosemary with Patchouli, Peppermint, Oregano, Myrrh, Melissa, Marjoram, Lavender, Helichrysum, Frankincense, Grounding Blend, Cypress, Clove, Cinnamon, Cassia, Calming Blend and Basil

Other Natural Methods of Treatment:

Think about essential oil-based supplements, such as Basic Vitality Supplements (LLV). Coconut oil is also known to improve cognitive performance and aid in problems with the brain, since it affects amyloid-b (Ab) which is a protein that causes degeneration. Every day, consume 2 teaspoons of organic cold-pressed, non-hydrogenated, and virgin coconut oil.

Circulation

Description:

Poor circulation occurs the result of blood flowing in a deficient manner that is noticeable in the legs, feet and hands, where the possibility of fatigue or cramps can be present. The problem with circulation can get worse and cause varicose veins, kidney problems and open ulcers, strokes, or slow wound healing. Good circulation also helps improve brain functioning.

Application:

To get immediate relief For immediate relief, dilute the essential oil in the appropriate amount (Cypress Massage Blend and Coriander Lemongrass along with a protective Blend are all suggested)

Apply the oil topically on the area affected. It is also possible to mix Frankincense Lemongrass, Cypress, and Marjoram in equal amounts dilute with carrier oil. Apply the mixture to the soles of feet as well as the heart.

Recommended oils:

Ylang Ylang, Sandalwood, Protective Blend, Peppermint, Myrrh, Massage Blend, Marjoram, Lemongrass, Lemon, Invigorating Blend, Ginger, Geranium, Frankincense, Eucalyptus, Cypress, Coriander, Black Pepper, and Basil

Other Natural Methods of Treatment:

Also , think about essential oil-based supplements such as these Basic Vitality Supplements (LLV) which can help with ongoing care for this condition. The active ingredient in garlic, allicin, aids in improving blood circulation. To get the most benefit consume 3- 4 Cloves of garlic every day in a stomach empty.

Common Brain-Aging Issues & Essential Oil Protocols

Normal aging does not result in severe dementia or memory loss, but they are the repercussions of certain neurodegenerative diseases like Alzheimer's. These diseases are the result of the accumulation of lipofuscin which creates plaques in the brain.

Other conditions that may cause neurodegeneration are infections, diabetes, as well as the use of certain medications which can trigger extreme confusion and delirium in older people. These conditions are not directly linked to brain function, but related to the diseases. Diabetes in particular can affect mental performance when blood sugar levels increase and fall in unison.

If you're confronted with changes in your behavior, thinking or memory that diverge from your normal routine or disrupt your daily tasks Get advice from your doctor to determine the root of the issue, and then aid in the treatment process by following the essential oil techniques listed below.

Essential Oil Protocols

Alzheimer's Disease

Description:

Alzheimer's disease causes the development of dementia, which can cause mood fluctuations as well as changes in social behaviour memory loss, and also the loss of brain functions that influence language abilities, judgement and social abilities. Alzheimer's disease is thought to be caused by the genetics of the disease, head injuries and chronic high blood pressure as well as aging, and new research has revealed nutritional deficiencies. The condition is progressive and can cause neurons to degenerate and gradually aggravate the symptoms. These include a slowing down, difficulties in multitasking, violent, or strange behavior, loss of things or objects, loss of interest, changes in sleeping patterns, as well as the inability to comprehend the world surrounding them.

Application:

* Cognitive impairment Dissolve your essential oil in accordance with the symptoms (Patchouli is recommended) and apply it topically to the brain stem as well as the soles of your feet. It is also possible to apply a drop of oil under the tongue.

* General health Dilute essential oils in the appropriate amount (Grounding Blend Melissa as well as Frankincense are all suggested) and apply it topically to the brain stem as well as the soles of your feet.

Recommended oils:

Ylang Ylang, Sandalwood, Rosemary with Patchouli, Peppermint, Oregano, Myrrh, Melissa, Marjoram, Lavender, Helichrysum, Frankincense, Grounding Blend, Cypress, Clove, Cinnamon, Cassia, Calming Blend and Basil

Other Natural Methods of Treatment:

Take a look at essential oil-based supplements, such as Basic Vitality Supplements (LLV). Coconut oil may also enhance cognitive performance and ease issues with the brain as it can influence amyloid-b (Ab) which is one of the components of the disease. Each day, you should consume 2 teaspoons of organic cold-pressed, non-hydrogenated and virgin coconut oil. Ginkgo biloba can also help ease anxiety, and increase memory and cognitive functioning. Each day, take one capsule of 120 mg daily divided into three doses.

Dementia

Description:

Dementia is a set of symptoms that occur in many different illnesses, which include memory loss, loss of judgment social skills, communication skills, as well as different brain processes. The cause of dementia is the aging process and illnesses such as MS and Huntington's disease. or other diseases that are associated with ageing, such as Alzheimer's. Other causes that cause dementia are nutrition deficiencies, alcoholism or brain inflammation, as well as tumors.

Application:

Basic treatment - dilute the chosen oil according to (Frankincense, Melissa, and Grounding Blend are all suggested) using an oil carrier and apply it topically to the neck's back around the brain stem twice times per day.

Oils to be recommended:

Ylang Ylang, Sandalwood, Rosemary (Patchouli), Peppermint, Oregano, Myrrh, Melissa, Marjoram, Lavender, Helichrysum, Grounding Blend, Geranium, Frankincense, Cypress, Clove, Cinnamon, Cassia, Calming Blend and Basil

Other Natural Methods of Treatment:

Think about essential oil-based supplements, such as Basic Vitality Supplements (LLV). Ginkgo biloba can help ease anxiety, and can increase memory and cognitive functioning. Every day , take a 120 mg capsule, divided into 3 doses.

Diabetes

Description:

Diabetes is a disease that results when glucose is not supplied to cells in the bloodstream. The sugar glucose is a byproduct in food items that, after being broken down, functions as fuel for fat liver cells, and muscle. The pancreas releases insulin which aids in the digestion of glucose. When the pancreas is not producing enough insulin the glucose cannot be absorbed and causes increased blood sugar. Some signs of diabetes include blurred vision and weight loss, as well as increased thirst and urination, tiredness, numbness and the sensation of tingling in feet. There are three types of diabetes: Type 1 (juvenile diabetes), Type 2 (most frequent form, usually caused by age, family history or physical inactivity) as well as gestational Diabetes (occurs during the pregnancy).

Application:

Type 2 - for application on the skin Massage the Grounding Blend into your feet each morning, and lavender at night. For use on the inside, pour 8-10 drops of your preferred essential oil (Basil or Coriander are recommended; add 2 drops of the Protective Blend to provide additional help) inside a capsule, and use it regularly.

Recommended oils:

Protection Blend, Peppermint, Marjoram Lavender, Helichrysum Grounding Blend, Geranium, Frankincense, Eucalyptus, Cypress, Coriander, Clove, Cinnamon, Cassia, and Basil

Other Natural Methods of Treatment:

Think about essential oils-based products such as Basic Vitality Supplements (LLV), Digestive Enzyme Complex, GI Cleansing Formula/Probiotic Defense Formula, as well as continuous Detoxification Blend. Make sure you are getting the right nutrition and weight loss through regular exercise and diet. Bitter gourds influence glucose metabolism, which aids in pancreatic insulin production. Every morning, remove the seeds from a couple of bitter gourds. Juice the fruit, add the juice to the water and then drink the bitter gourd juice prior to eating.

Nerve Damage

Description:

Damage to the nerves can be the result of a range of conditions, including autoimmune diseases, IBD, multiple sclerosis or diabetes, ALS or Lupus. It may also be caused by infection (Lyme, Hepatitis, HIV) as well as cancerous growths, treatments for cancer medications or toxins, arthritis pressure or trauma, as well as various other problems. In the end, symptoms can vary based on the cause and can be accompanied by sensory impairment (dizziness and discomfort, tingling, numbness burning) as well as motor damage (paralysis and weakening, twitching, or muscle atrophy) as well as autoimmune-related damage (constipation dry eyes, dry mouth problems with bladders, sexual dysfunction and excessive sweating).

Application:

To heal damaged nerves, ease the pain, improve circulation and guard against infection blend 15 drops Geranium 10 drops each of Wintergreen and Helichrysum eight drops Marjoram, 6 drops Cypress five drops peppermint and 2 drops each of Lemon and Clove in a small glass bottle or container. Mix well and dilute 3-4 drops using an oil carrier and apply it topically on the an affected area for at least three times per day.

Recommended oils:

Vetiver, Roman Chamomile, Peppermint Patchouli, Massage Blend, Marjoram, Oregano, Lemongrass, Lemon, Lavender, Juniper Helichrysum Grounding Blend, Grapefruit, Geranium Cypress Cassia and Birch

Other Natural Methods of Treatment:

Apply a warm , padded compress to the area affected for 5-7 minutes to alleviate numbness or discomfort.

Neuropathy

Description:

Neuropathy (or peripheral neuropathy) is in the case that your peripheral nerve system gets damaged due to infections as well as malnutrition, toxins or trauma, or other conditions such as diabetes. The condition can manifest in a variety of forms, including carpel tunnel syndrome. It typically involves feeling of being numb, muscles control, loss of numbness burning or tingling.

Application:

To treat neuropathy in the feet, apply 2 to 4 drops of the Grounding Blend into the feet. Then, blend two drops each with Marjoram, Cypress, and Basil and massage into your feet. Add 2-4 drops of peppermint Then apply the hot compress.

Check out other protocols as per the their underlying conditions.

Oils to be recommended:

Peppermint Marjoram and Grounding Blend Cypress And Basil

Other Natural Methods of Treatment:

Take a supplement of 100 milligrams of vitamin B-1 each day. Apply cayenne cream to the area affected to alleviate the pain caused by neuropathy.

Parkinson's Disease

Description:

Parkinson's disease is a prevalent nervous system disorder that manifests due to a deficiency of dopamine reaching into the part of the brain that regulates movement of the body, resulting in shakes, tremors, and difficulty walking. Parkinson's disease is a progressive disorder and is often seen in people who are over 50 years old. Initial symptoms include trembling and an ache in the legs and a lack of facial expression. Advanced symptoms include constipation, drooling difficulties with mobility, more muscles pain as well as dementia, depression and anxiety.

Application:

For an internal application, place 2-3 drops Frankincense beneath the tongue. Apply topically Frankincense on the top of the head as well as the base of the skull as well as the spine. Also, dilute your selected oil according to the recommended dosage (Wild Orange Tea Tree and Grounding Blend and Protective Blend Lavender Peppermint, Massage Blend, or Soothing Blend are recommended) using an oil carrier and employing the Massage Blend method, apply directly to the area.

Recommended oils:

Ylang Ylang, Wild Orange, Peppermint, Myrrh, Lavender and grounding Blend, Ginger, Frankincense Cypress, Basil, and

Other Natural Methods of Treatment:

Think about essential oil-based products such as Basic Vitality Supplements (LLV), GI Cleansing Formula, and Probiotic Defense Formula. To improve mental clarity keep a balanced diet and lifestyle. Fish oil is high in omega-3 acids. It helps boost the production of hormones and nerve tissue health and brain function. To determine the right dosage of supplements made from fish oil, talk to your physician.

Stroke

Description:

Strokes can occur when a region of the brain doesn't get enough blood due to the blockage of blood vessels or bleeding from the brain. This causes brain cells to die within a matter of minutes. Signs of strokes are difficulties speaking and headaches, as well as anxiety, walking difficulties or standing and numbness or paralysis or tingling on one part that is affected, mainly in the arm or face. Strokes may occur due to hemorrhaging (damage to the blood vessel in the brain) as well as Ischemic (blockage of blood flow) or a temporary ischemic attacks (mini-stroke where blood flow is restricted for a short time, but it returns).

Application:

General recovery - After seeking medical attention, follow an internal application regimen consisting of 1-2 drops Frankincense on the tongue twice a every day. Couple this with a topically applied application of Massage Blend to the part in the middle of your heart.

Recommended oils:

Ylang Ylang, Peppermint, Melissa massage Blend, Lavender, Helichrysum and Blend for Grounding Blend, Grapefruit, Frankincense, Cypress, and Basil

Other Natural Methods of Treatment:

Think about essential oil-based supplements, such as Basic Vitality Supplements (LLV). If you experience stroke, you should seek medical attention immediately. To decrease the risk of having a stroke, adopt healthy habits - that is to you should exercise regularly, eat a healthy diet and limit your the consumption of alcohol, don't smoke, manage your blood pressure and control stress.

Chapter 15: Reducing Wrinkles Tips

When it comes to reducing wrinkles, you must take your time and consider your choices seriously. There are plenty of factors that can be involved in the health and wellbeing of your skin. It is often difficult to comprehend the reasons why these products don't work, even when they promise ways to make it happen and the ways in which they operate. If you're thinking about wrinkle creams or the regimen of facelifts you may end up breaking your bank when you do it. You should think about going through a procedure to determine the most efficient option for your requirements before doing any of those.

The first thing you should think about is the health of your skin. Your skin should be healthy for you to keep it from getting old. It will also make you appear healthy and slim. If you're suffering from lines does not mean that your skin is unhealthy. Actually, it suggests that you should be more attentive to your overall health. The best place to start is to start with your diet.

* Do you have the ability to eat healthy food items, such as an eating plan that is rich in high-color vegetables?

* Do you consume a lot of food items that aren't balanced for you?

* Would you like to eat food which are extremely oily?

Many of these issues could make a number of parts of your body to function in the proper way. If you are considering buying treatments for wrinkles, begin by improving your general diet. This means that you provide your body with the necessary nutrients via the foods you consume. Many people make the error of believing that what they consume doesn't matter. If you're beginning to notice wrinkles early on they could be caused because of a lack of appropriate diet. Enhance your diet and your overall health and your skin's appearance.

Reduced Wrinkles: Stay Clear Of The Sun

Check out your approach to taking care of your skin before buying the most costly wrinkle cream. No matter what treatment you're planning to use it, if you're not looking at your skin in the beginning, it won't fulfill your needs. Many people are guilty of applying a wrinkle cream an emergency bandage, but if you don't address the problem first. However, that band aid will not be effective. Butbefore you do that, you need take a look at your current situation.

Many people have lines due to the influence of sun's rays. The sun's rays can be fatal to our body. For some who wear sunscreen is only an option in the past when the beach is the spot or when temperatures are at their peak. However, during cloudy days or the winter months ultraviolet sun's rays are shining through, damaging your skin. The more exposure you are exposed to, the more likely you'll require action to repair it. Not only are UV radiations the most common cause for skin cancer, but they are also the reason to wrinkles, too.

So, what do you do? Consider looking for items that offer UV protection. Apply sunscreen to your skin prior to applying other products. Be sure that when you leave your home each day, you do similar to your children. It is a fact that your skin needs to be protected with sunscreen if are planning to appear older or younger. If you don't apply it , or don't use regularly enough, the possibility of getting sun damage lines and wrinkles are a component of the offer. Do not let your skin be affected by these issues. Stop wrinkles from appearing by using sunscreen.

The reduction of wrinkles: options to Take into

If you've made an initiative to boost your overall health and well-being The next step on the path is improving the condition of your skin by other methods. There are many other options available in the market that could either significantly or in a minimal way reduce the appearance of lines and improve the appearance of your skin. All of these options worked for a couple of people, but it's not guaranteed that any treatment will work for you. Discussing your cosmetic surgeon and doctor is the best way to determine your benefits.

Here are some options.

* Creams to reduce wrinkles. They are abundant and definitely can help. If you want to ensure that you purchase one that will be useful you should look for ones with Retinal. The label should state that or should claim they have Vitamin E, Vitamin C as well as Vitamin A. Things that promise to be miraculous products won't actually very beneficial, but.

* Botox. It's among the most known products for eliminating wrinkles on the face. Here's the ideal solution for you if you are thinking of seeking a solution that isn't overly and not invasive. Be aware that you may have to get it redesigned frequently. It's a task that can be

completed in your lunch break and is a simple choice.

The face lift. It doesn't need to be, though it's a more severe option. There are a variety of smaller types of changes that could be implemented to improve the appearance of your skin. attractive. Small and big changes could be implemented to eliminate the wrinkles in your skin.

Skin Care for sensitive skin

There are a few basic rules that govern "Sensitive Skin Care". Before we get into the guidelines for gentle skincare, it is crucial to know what makes an extremely sensitive skin. Skin that is delicate is the kind that can't take on any unpleasant conditions (ecological/other) and often gets angry when connected to unusual products (including cosmetics). Due to this, certain products are labeled as sensitive skincare products. Their awareness of the products may however differ from person to the individual (and depending on this the gentle skincare techniques differ too).

All types of skin react negatively to chemicals and liquids. But, the damage begins typically after a specific threshold (or threshold). This threshold is extremely sensitive for those with delicate skin and results in skin getting damaged quickly and easily. Skincare products that are delicate keep their level at an acceptable level or even ward off the possibility of toxin.

Below are a few methods for caring for sensitive skin:

* Use skincare products that are gentle only (i.e. The products that are specifically designed to be used for sensitive skin only). Also, read the instructions or notes on the product to identify if there are any particular restrictions or warnings that relate to the product).

* Additionally, in the list of products for delicate skin choose the one that is free of preservatives, colors and other chemicals.

* Don't use toners.

It is possible to put cotton gloves beneath the rubber gloves in case you are going to be allergic to plastic.

A different important tip for "sensitive skin care' is to stay away from excessive exposure to sunlight. Make sure to apply sunscreen before venturing in the sunlight.

Avoiding contact with dirt contaminants can be vital for the care of sensitive skin. So, make sure to protect yourself adequately prior to leaving.

* Make sure you use hypoallergenic, noncomedogenic moisturizers similar to a delicate skincare item (when there's no such thing described as a delicate skincare product)

* Use soap alcohol or soaps that are free. After going out in the sun, wash your face.

* Exfoliate a lot or do not wash. It can cause reddishness and even an irritation.

* Do not keep your makeup put on an excessive amount of time.

Skin Care Products that fight the signs of aging

"Anti-aging skin care" is a common concept in the present day. Everyone wants to reduce their age with anti-aging skincare techniques (along with several people are also effective). However, anti-aging skincare can't be achieved through any magical potion. The process of aging can be slowed down by anti-aging skincare. Here are some methods to combat the signs of aging:

1. Follow a healthy eating plan A balanced and healthy diet can be the most important factor to maintaining the body's metabolism in good shape. Consume plenty of fruit and vegetables (natural) They're the most potent source of fiber, and have an extremely refreshing effect on your body. Avoid eating fatty and oily foods and drinks; they not only are deficient in essential vitamins, but they also lead to obesity and various diseases that can slow the aging process.

2. Beat stress: It is the most effective anti-aging skin care measure. The metabolism of your body affects it and accelerates ageing. Relaxation, a relaxing shower and exercise are excellent ways to beat tension. Aromatherapy is a method to ease the pressure.

3. Drink plenty of fluids Anti-aging skin care can't be more simple than this. Water aids in making it less prone to illness and helps eliminate toxins from the body, thereby maintaining its health. About eight cups of drinking liquid (daily) is the preferred choice of doctors of all kinds.

4. Regular exercise is an effective anti-aging process for skincare. It helps in cleansing your skin, eliminating contaminants that come with the exercise, in addition to tightening the muscle tissue. The exercise should be followed by an energizing bath in order to completely rid the body of contaminants.

5. Avoid the use of strong chemicals in your skin. Products for your skin that are organic are a good alternative. Making use

of natural skincare items (homemade or commercial) could be a beneficial anti-aging method.

6. Don't overuse skincare products. Extremely and dangerous software are both dangerous.

7. Be aware of skin problems and it could lead to lasting skin damage. Take a look at over-the-counter remedies and then consult your doctor and seek the advice of your physician if that does not work.

However, they do appear to rapidly oxidize (making the risk for skin). Keep them. If the color turns yellowish-brown, it signifies that vitamin D has been oxidized and the product is no better to use.

9. Make sure your skin is protected from ultraviolet radiation; ultra violet light is known as accelerating ageing. So, a good sunscreen product should be a an integral part of your anti-aging skin care regimen.

Herbal Skin Care

The topic of skincare isn't a hot one in modern times, it's been around since the beginning of time which was when the natural approach to skin health was likely the only method to take care of skin during the course of. However, modern skincare has transformed to a massive extent. The use of synthetic or chemical ingredients has replaced natural, organic skincare regimens.

The organic recipes for skincare that used to be commonplace aren't the same anymore (and they're also not known to large numbers of people). The shift from natural skincare to chemical-based, could result from a couple of factors - our lack of activity (or just the rapid pace of our lives) and also the increasing commercialization of skin care.

The professional skincare products have to be paired with ingredients to increase their shelf lives, giving them a greater power in comparison to the clean products that are made at home.

It appears that things are quickly changing and more people are opting for organic and natural skincare products. Yet, there is no desire to ensure that they are at home, and thus the demand for industrial skincare products is growing.

What exactly are the natural ingredients in skincare, or herbs?

The new aloe Vera is an unadulterated hydrant that aids in soothing the skin. It also aids in healing sunburns and cuts.

A variety of herbs are believed as having cleaning properties. Dandelion, lime flowers, and rosemary are some of these cleansers. Their natural skin-care properties are activated when they are used with other herbs, such as tea

Antiseptics are a different important part in Organic skincare. Thyme and lavender are examples of plants that are believed to have antiseptic properties.

Tea is an essential ingredient in the natural skin care.

Natural oils that are made from plant ingredients offer a different method of natural skin care. Tea tree oil, rose oil borage oil, primrose oil are just a few commonly used oils in natural skincare.

Aromatherapies and holistic treatments fall under the skin care treatments that are natural.

Organic skincare is beneficial not just for keeping your skin healthy, but also for treating skin problems such as eczema and psoriasis. Natural skincare products aren't known to cause any adverse results (the principal reason to choose these products over synthetic ones) Furthermore organic skincare products can be made quickly at home, which makes them much more attractive. Thus, natural skincare may be the way to go.

This doesn't mean that you should completely remove the synthetic items. A lot of people are aware of speaking with their physician in the event that he recommends a synthetic product. It is essential to acknowledge that certain skin care instructions may require the use of scientifically-proven products for skincare that are natural and low-cost.

Chapter 16: Quinoa

If you've visited the healthiest restaurant and ordered salad, you may have noticed tiny yellow balls that were rather intriguing. They are what people are talking about. They're the superfood referred to as the quinoa. The word quinoa actually is "mother of grains" and it's not without reason. In people of the Incas it was considered to be sacred as it gave longevity for those who consumed it. People believed in health benefits of this food, and made it a main product in their diet.

However, this superfood isn't actually one of the grains. Actually it is more similar to spinach and beets than oatmeal. It is , however, far better than any of them in terms of nutrition.

Important nutrients in Quinoa

* Protein

* Fiber

* Vitamin A, E

* Calcium

* Potassium

* Iron

* Phosphorus

* Manganese

* Zinc

* Copper

* Magnesium

* Riboflavin

* Tyrosine

* Lysine

Anti-Ageing Properties of Quinoa

Skin that is firmer The most important of the nutrients that are found in Quinoa is the amino acid lysine. It's known to stimulate an increase in collagen production and the production of elastin that keep skin smooth and looking youthful.

Skin that is soft It is because the riboflavin present in Quinoa makes the skin soft and soft and smooth. It also reduces the appearance of fine lines.

Evens out skin tone If you've got marks on the face, or discolorationon your skin, the different vitamins contained in the quinoa help bring out the skin's color.

Reduces the risk of breakouts -If you believe your face is oily try taking some quinoa and observe how it can help you combat acne.

Improves skin health faster Lysine found in quinoa treats damaged skin tissues and cells, and helps in repairing and healing them quicker. This is a great option for healing when you've just had surgery or suffered an injury.

Hair that is stronger It is because of certain amino acids found in quinoa which ensure that the hair shaft is healthy and strong. These amino acids can restore hair that's been damaged. Vitamin E also regulates the production of oil so that hair strands won't break when they become tangled.

Hair that is thicker If you're worried about hair loss look into the quinoa. It helps nourish hair follicles and stimulates hair growth.

No more split endsBecause quinoa is rich in protein, it can prevent the growth of split ends, by making hair more flexible.

Don't worry about dandruff anymore. If it's always a mess on your scalp, incorporating quinoa into the of your daily diet is an ideal choice for you. The minerals in quinoa such as iron, calcium and phosphorus will keep your scalp from becoming dry and flaky.

Reduces the appearance of grey hair Quinoa is a source of tyrosine. This helps to maintain the natural coloration of hair.

Prevents diabetes -- Since the quinoa plant is high in healthy carbohydrates It controls blood sugar in a healthy way. This lowers the chance of developing diabetes, and helps keep blood sugar levels under control in the event that you already have diabetes.

Helps prevent migraines. Migraines can be very painful experience. Because quinoa contains high levels of riboflavin, it helps to promote regular blood flow to the brain. This stops migraines from occurring.

There is no gluten, even though it's technically not a cereal, quinoa is a good choice as an alternative to grains that is gluten-free.

Lose weight Quinoa is low in fat , and it helps you feel fuller for longer time. When you are exercising and eating right Quinoa is a superfood that makes it easy to shed weight.

Promotes digestion -- Say goodbye to constipation. Due to the high amount of dietary fiber in Quinoa, your digestive health will be improved while your stool movements could occur regularly.

Cleans the arteries -- One of the numerous wonders that quinoa can perform, some can help prevent cardiovascular diseases and strokes.

Enhance athletic performance Warriors long ago consumed this superfood for increases in stamina, energy as well as strength and muscle repair.

How Do I Use Quinoa

If you purchase Quinoa seeds, make sure to keep them in a location that has no moisture, and in a container that air can't get into.

Quinoa's most popular form isn't a powder as many other superfoods. This is the place the perfect opportunity to unleash your creative juices. There are a variety of ways to cook quinoa and it can enhance the flavor of your food.

The flavor of this superfood has been described as sweet and nutty. If cooked, it provides an excellent texture and is very chewy.

In preparing quinoa seeds first you must get rid of the outer layer. If you don't do this, you could experience stomach discomfort after eating the seeds. Clean the quinoa first and after that, for 2 hours, soak them in the water. Refresh the water, rinse and soak until the foam has gone.

You can now cook quinoa the same way as it was any other grain. You have the option of baking, grinding, cooking or frying them. You can then cook quinoa similar to other grains.

Chapter 17: Healthy Eating and being healthy

There are certain food items - nuts, fruits, vegetables and lentils, that are acknowledged as having anti antioxidant nutrients. Food is an essential part of the quality of life. But it is vital to consume proper quantities of food to get the greatest results in our quest to keep youthfulness.

Limit the quantity of meals you consume during meals. Researchers of St Paul's University discovered that decreasing the calories consumed also decreased the production of the thyroid hormone T3 that is linked to slowing down the metabolism process. They believe that a lower level of T3 levels in the body can aid in slowing the process of aging.

It is crucial to be aware of your weight and figures. Make sure you are maintaining the correct Body Mass Index (BMI) for your weight and height.

A healthy body shape helps to keep a youthful appearance.

To preserve our youth and slow the aging process our bodies, we should eat a greater amount of fruits, vegetables , and nuts. It is recommended to consume fruits and vegetables of all shades as they all have the same amount of antioxidants.

Antioxidants combat free radicals that cause harm to the cells in the body. Free radicals are typically produced in the process of oxidation within the body. They are the result of transformation of oxygen and food to energy.

People who reside in the islands in Okinawa, Japan who are one of the oldest people on earth consume more plants and fish.

Consume greater amounts of Omega H3fatty acids that are found in walnuts and sardines . Omega 3 helps to maintain a healthy, radiant skin, aids in stabilizing the mood, strengthens bones and decreases inflammation, all of which aid in extending youthfulness.

Below is a list of foods - NUTS, VEGETABLES FRUITS, LENTILS AND FRUITS THAT have been recognized as having anti-aging nutrients and properties.

I will discuss each as well as the characteristics and nature of the work they perform within the human body to slow the process of aging.

Nuts

Nuts are a rich source of protein and good fats as well as omega 3 essential fats. They aid in regulating cholesterol levels in the body, and improve brain function. This assists in preventing the effects of aging on the brain, such as memory loss or forgetfulness.

Walnuts Pecans cashews, almonds, and walnuts are just a few options of nuts available that fall under this class. Although they are high in calories, nuts provide excellent nutritional benefits to the body, and are the perfect snack. For optimal health be sure to eat the nuts in their natural state without salt.

Fruits

Fruits contain a great deal of antioxidants. These antioxidants aid in fighting free radicals, which can cause damage to cells in the body. Through their antioxidant effects fruits can help in reducing the negative effects of age. Here are some of the most important fruits:

Tomato

Tomato is a great food. It decreases the likelihood of developing cardiovascular illnesses and also slows down the growth of inflammation. Consuming tomatoes is beneficial in fighting cancers such as stomach, pancreatic, lung and the esophageal cancer. In addition, tomatoes contain the powerful antioxidant the lycopene that fights the degenerative diseases that generally appear as we age.

Papaya

Papaya is a must for skin. The fruit is natural skin toner that fights the development of wrinkles, aiding in keeping the body young.

Apple

Apple is a rich source of quercetin, catechins chlorogenic acid, and phloridzin. They are all powerful antioxidants, which fight against diseases like prostate and lung cancers. Apple helps reduce the risk of suffering from alzheimer's disease. It assists keep the skin fresh and healthy since it helps in the maintenance of healthy levels of water in the skin.

Blueberry

Blueberry contains about five kinds of anthocyanins that are powerful antioxidants. The large amount of antioxidants helps in preventing and limiting the decline of the brain that happens in old age. They assist in maintaining collagen that keeps your skin looking smooth and free of wrinkles, thus helping to prevent some signs of ageing.

This helps keep the skin looking fresh. Blueberry is a great source of antioxidants, more than other superfoods.

Blackberry

The primary role of blackberry to support the ability to live longer is its ability to increase bone density.

Raspberry

Raspberry is a great source of vitamin C and antioxidants. They can fight cancer and can aid in treating high blood pressure because they help reduce the levels of cholesterol that are high.

Grape

Grapes are rich in manganese as well as Vitamin C. These substances help protect against the harmful consequences caused by Ultra Violet Radiation resulting from direct sunlight that hits the skin. The antioxidants' actions assist in slowing the process of aging.

Cherry

Cherry is very efficient in fighting against the process of aging. Cherry aids in reducing arthritic pain, which is usually seen in the later years of age, decrease cholesterol levels and reduce inflammation that can manifest as a sign of old age.

Avocado

The Avocado pear has a high quantity of Potassium, Vitamin B complex as well as Vitamin C. Additionally, it also contains a substance called Glutathione that reduces the effects of the aging process. Avocado is extremely nourishing to your skin and keeps it moisturized and well-hydrated.

Kiwi Fruit

The Kiwi fruit that is green in appearance, has a wealth of antioxidants. The Kiwi fruit aids in firming the skin and combat wrinkles. Kiwi reduces the chance of blood clots, blood lipids , and reduces constipation.

The kiwi fruit contains about twice the amount of vitamin C in oranges, and it can decrease inflammation. All of these can help reduce the negative effects of aging.

Pineapple

Pineapple is a rich source of vitamin C as well as bromelain, a compound. It helps reduce inflammation and slows the growth of arthritis as well as joint pain.

Pomegranate

Pomegranate has riboflavin, phosphorus as well as a variety of vitamins and minerals that aid in maintaining flexibility and firmness the skin through the increase of the collagen. Additionally, it contains enzymes that assist in lowering the concentrations of blood sugar and cholesterol. It also lowers the risk of developing prostate cancer. It also helps fight premature aging by shielding your skin from the damaging UV rays of the sun.

Mangosteen

Mangosteen contains a significant amount of vitamin C and catechin, which can be powerful antioxidants which protect against cell damage due to actions that free radicals perform. It also provides skin with a soft and radiant glow.

Goji Berry

Goji berries contain 500 more vitamin C per gram than orange. Goji berries are packed with huge amounts of carotenoids. It promotes the quality of sleep, improves the libido and memory, decreases fat and aids in making us look younger.

Watermelon

It is packed with a lot of vitamins, minerals , and antioxidants. It shields skin from sunburn while keeping it well-nourished and preventing wrinkles and discoloration that are often indications of ageing.

Vegetables

Vegetables are a rich source of minerals and vitamins that are essential to the body. They also contain antioxidants which assist in combating the harmful negative effects of free radicals, which damage the cells in the body. It is recommended to consume a large amount of vegetables along with drinking plenty of fluids. When your stomach is full with vegetables and water there is no any room for junk food and the sugary fizzy sodas. It is a good idea to eat as many kinds and varieties of vegetables as you can, particularly those that are green and leafy.

Eat these vegetables frequently will allow you keep looking younger

Cabbage

Cabbage is loaded with cancer fighting nutrients than other vegetables. Cabbage can fight some types of cancer, such as prostate colon, ovarian, and breast cancers. It is packed with lots of vitamin C as well as calcium and fiber, including the compound Indoles which aids in lowering blood pressure. Cabbage can also help combat blood clotting and aids in the efficient treatment of wounds.

Sweet Potatoes

Sweet potatoes are loaded with lots of carotene vitamin C as well as calcium and potassium that can help reduce stroke risk and combat cancer. Carotene is a component that assists in protecting against blurred vision and cataracts.

Butternut Squash

Butternut squash has a good amount of vitamin A as well as C. It also has Niacin and potassium. It can reduce the risk of wrinkles, enhances night vision, and helps to stabilize your cardiovascular system.

Kale

Kale contains a large amount of vitamins B, A as well as C. It assists in establishing bones and shields eyes from the harmful Ultra Violet Rays of the sun.

Cauliflower

Cauliflower aids in battling the growth of prostate and breast cancer. It's a source of the chemical allicin that helps maintain healthy heart health. It also helps in the detoxification of liver and blood. It also has a significant content of vitamin C

Carrot

Carrots are rich in Vitamins A, B and C as well as potassium sodium and calcium. Carrots have a high amount of beta carotene that fights cataract and protects DNA.

Arugula

Arugula has beta-carotene and lots of vitamin C and folic acid potassium, and fiber. It aids in maintaining healthy heart health, good eye health , and decreases the chance of fractures by increasing bone density.

Broccoli

Broccoli is a rich source of antioxidants, as well as Vitamins B6, C, and E. It decreases the chance of developing gastric, breast colon, prostate, and pancreatic tumors. It also helps prevent brain injury and the detrimental consequences of diabetes.

Spinach

Spinach is a rich source of vitamins B, A C, D and K . It improves mental alertness and reduces the risk of various cancers such as colon, ovarian and liver, as well as prostate.

Red Pepper

Red pepper can help keep healthy skin and cardiovascular health. It decreases the chance of developing ovarian, lung cervical, and prostate cancers.

Mushroom

Mushroom can reduce the risk of colon and prostate cancers. It can help lower blood pressure and also helps to enhance the body's natural detoxification system.

Lentils

Lentils are legumes, and they is believed to have been around as long as the man on the planet. Lentils are edible, and nutritious. There are black, red and brown lentils, such as kidney beans, black-eyed beans along with soya beans. It appears that each country has its own distinct variety of lentils, but they all share the same components.

Care of Cardiovascular System

Lentils aid in digestion when eaten frequently because of the large amount of fibers in the diet that they have. They are a good source of protein and a small amount of fat. The presence of moderate amounts of magnesium help maintain the cardiovascular system's suppleness and helps to reduce blood pressure. These are common conditions related to the aging process.

Muscle Regeneration

Sprouted lentils have the potent amino acids - methionine as well as cysteine which aid in the regeneration of muscles and overall maintenance in the general health of our bodies. This can be beneficial for those who are elderly and see a reduction in the muscle mass they have as they age.

Cells and Gene Maintenance

The antioxidants in lentils fight free radicals that usually harm cells and the genes of the body. This can lead to premature ageing.

Improve Brain Function

Vitamins and minerals in lentils can help keep the brain in top shape. This can help fight the decline of brain functions that can lead to dementia and memory loss that usually develops during old age.

Lentils contain vitamin B3, which aids in maintaining the nervous and digestive systems.

Lentils can also be used to combat the development of alzheimer's disease and cataracts that usually occur in the later years of age.

Beware of lentils

Ingestion of excess amounts of protein could cause damage to the kidneys. This is due to the fact that the kidney is stressed when it tries to eliminate the excess protein.

Multivitamins

While a balanced diet must include a mix of moderate portions of protein, carbohydrate, along with healthy fats there are times when the body isn't capable of getting the complete supply of vitamins, minerals , and other nutrients. To overcome these deficiencies, it's advised to buy a excellent multivitamins. There are many firms that specialize in geriatric health have high-quality multivitamins designed specifically for seniors.

Chapter 18: Anti-Aging Drinks Recipes

for radiant skin and glowing health

Juice, smoothies and tea recipes to slow the process of aging

It is well-known that ageing is a natural thing but perhaps we aren't aware that there are a variety of methods to slow down the process. You are what you eat , and your body's body will reflect exactly the food you consume as fuel. If you are living a unhealthy lifestyle , be sure that your aging process is faster and eventually you awake in 40s that look like 50s or more. Anti-aging refers to the slowing down and reverse ageing process. It can play a huge part in the length as well as the quality. You only need to know the best way to achieve this and then take action to transform your way of life.

Make-me-glow Berry Smoothie

Cup of mix Berries

One cup Greek Yogurt

1 teaspoon. raw honey

1 teaspoon. coconut oil

1/3 1 teaspoon. Bee pollen powder (don't use it if are allergic to)

Crushed Ice

Combine the ingredients together in a blender, and serve.

They are high in antioxidants that fight free radicals and hinder the process of aging. Blueberries blackberries, raspberries and Huckleberries - they are popular throughout North of America.

Bee pollen is a rich source of proteins from animal sources. It has more amino acids than eggs, beef, and cheese that weigh the same. It can be utilized as an energy booster as well as a as a skin-soother (regeneration of cells) as well as for the treatment of allergies, to boost the immune system and for fertility issues.

Rooibos as well as Cardamom Iced Tea

3 Rooibos tea bags

3 crushed cardamom pods

1 teaspoon. lemon juice

1 teaspoon. raw honey

Boil one cup of water and add 3 crushed cardamom seeds. Add 3 tea bags one teaspoon. lemon juice and 1 teaspoon. Raw honey into a cup , and put the tea through the strainer. Take tea bags out when the tea has cooled and cool it down.

Rooibos is an South African anti-aging secret that has been utilized for centuries to combat the signs of aging. It contains a high level of antioxidants and some of them have anti-mutagenic properties, preventing cancers.it can also protects you against Parkinsons/Alzheimers disease and can relieve the skin conditions.

Cardamom is a spice for anti-aging which is loaded with a lot of antioxidants. They help to boost the immune system, and also protect the body from the effects of aging.

Age defying C-juice

1 Guava

Half cup of juice from oranges

1 kiwi

Parsley clumps

5-6 raisins

Combine them all in a blender, and you'll have the most delicious and healthy juice.

Guava, parsley, Kiwi and orange are not just tasty and nutritious, they are they are also excellent natural ingredients for skin treatment. They are packed with skin-nourishing nutrients, including Vitamin C and E as well as antioxidants that are vital for improving the health of your skin. They also aid in the regeneration of skin cells and the production of collagen, which makes the skin more elastic and youthful.

Magic juices of hibiscus and rose

1 Tbsp. dried rose petals

1 tablespoon. dried hibiscus petals

Three slices of lemon

1 teaspoon. raw honey

A little cardamom powder

Ice cubes

Make 2 cups of water together with rose petals cardamom powder and hibiscus petals and allow it to boil for five minutes. Then strain the water, then add sugar or honey and put it in the refrigerator and serve chilled served with slices of lemon or frozen cubes.

You may not know that it is known as"the "Natural Botox plant". It is a cult favorite in the field of skin care due to the fact that it is an alpha-hydroxy natural ingredient. acids. It aids in exfoliating the skin and speeds up cell turnover, and controlling acne. The reason this plant is referred to as the Botox plant is that it boosts the amount of moisture and increases the elasticity and flexibility that the skin.

Rose is one of the most effective anti-aging ingredient. It is able to rejuvenate and revitalize skin by eliminating dead skin cells, and provide an appearance and glow to aged skin.

Date and cacao smoothie

1 cup coconut milk

1 Tbsp. cacao powder

1tsp. flax seeds

1 teaspoon. chia seeds

3 dates pitted and soaked in water for around an hour

1 teaspoon. Maca root powder

Five to six drops vanilla

Crushed Ice

Blend all ingredients in a blender and serve.

The recipe is packed with incredible ingredients like cacao and flax, chia dates, maca, and cacao.

Cacao beans contain natural chemical known as flavonoids, a kind of antioxidant compound that improves general health and reduces the chance of getting sick.

Personally, I've never had the pleasure of trying Chia seeds, but I do know that the early Aztecs collected chia seeds of the Salvia hispanica plant and they used as the primary food source for centuries. The seeds were given to their gods, and used for rituals. It also served to exchange currency. Aztecs warriors used it for power and energy.

Chia seeds are rich in healthy oils, antioxidants, proteins as well as fibers, vitamins and minerals.

It is loaded with magnesium, iron, Omega 3, copper vitamin B zinc, calcium, potassium, and phosphorus. Chia seeds have some of the best anti-aging substances and you'll feel the benefits after you add Chia seeds to your diet.

The three components that power flaseed-omega3: lignans, antioxidants assist in restoring the elasticity of skin as well as concealing wrinkles and reversing the signs of ageing. They also help hydrate skin and diminish the appearance of wrinkles, fine lines and dullness.

Maca is the mystery of Peru. It is high in iron, calcium and vitamin C, as well as essential amino acids. It is important to note that, as the Incas were aware of, is that maca has amazing rejuvenating abilities.

Tropical Beauty

Half cup of papaya

1 cup pineapple

1 cup coconut milk

1 Tbsp. hemp seed powder

1 cup mango cubes

5-6 soaked raisins

Blend them together before serving the delectable product.

Papaya: the vibrant orange-pink shade of papaya signifies that it's awash in carotenoids that fight cancer. It's a great source of carotene Vitamin C, carotene, important minerals, and papain. It's an effective exfoliant and moisturizer and helps reduce signs of age-related spots.

The fruit is rich in vitamin C as well as bromelain, which can be used as an effective acne treatment. Bromelain is an enzyme which soothes the skin . It has also been utilized for centuries across South as well as Central America to fight inflammation. Consuming pineapple juice can help the body produce collagen and amino acids, which aid in tissue and cell repair.

Hemp seeds have a beneficial anti-inflammatory ratio 3:1 of omega-6 to omega-3 fat. It has a beneficial form of omega-6 fat known as GLA(GLA, gamma linolenic acid).

GLA aids in metabolism, aids in the process of burning fat, and helps to maintain skin health. It reduces the risk to develop inflammation.

Mango is often referred to as a superfruit because it has high levels of Vitamin A as well as vitamin C. It is essential in aiding in the creation of collagen protein as well as the maintenance of blood vessels. This reduces the ageing processes of skin. It also aids in boosting the immune system of the body, to ensure the health of the brain and decrease blood pressure.

Exotic beauty potion

1 cup coconut milk

1 ripe peach

5-6 drops vanilla extract

1/3rd teaspoon. Pure pearl powder

1 TSP. fresh rose petals

1 teaspoon. Manuka honey

Crushed Ice

Blend all the ingredients in a blender, and then enjoy this healthy cup!

Coconut milk helps reduce wrinkles through promoting collagen production and repair.

Peach aids in maintaining body's skin, bones, a healthy nervous system and a healthy eye. Peaches are a symbol of the longevity of life and in immortality for China. The peaches and their pulp of peaches contain antioxidants such as beta-crytoxanthin and zeaxanthin which protects the body from illnesses. It is rich in phenolic as well as carothenoid substances that possess anti-tumor and anti-cancer properties.

Pearl powder is the most popular Chinese beauty secret that was utilized by royalty in China hundreds of years ago to maintain their skin's perfect and radiant.

Benefits of pearl powder:

Softens and firm youthful, glowing skin

Promotes new skin growth

Regenerates collagen

Reduces the appearance of aging skin

Reduces fine lines, wrinkles, sagging

Enhances the elasticity of skin

Repairs damaged skin from sun damage and scars

Minimizes large pores

The rose petals that are used in cosmetic formulations can reduce the effects of ultraviolet light as well as other environmental stressors that could result in premature aging of the skin.

Manuka honey is an amazing food that has the potential to be an anti-aging and powerful agent.

Vanilla, an exotic ingredient can give the impression of freshness and beauty. It helps to tighten the pores and shields against the imperfections on the skin.

The combination of orange and saffron is a great revitalizer.

2 cups of water

5-6 strands of saffron

1/3 of an ounce. (10 grams.) dried orange peel

A little the spice nutmeg

1 teaspoon. organic raw honey

You can crush ice if wish for it to be served cold

Boil 2 cups of water the dried peel of an orange, saffron, and Nutmeg powder. It should boil for 5 to 6 minutes. Add honey to it to serve hot. You can also keep it refrigerated and serve with a bit of ice for those who prefer it cold.

Saffron is extensively used throughout Middle East, Asia and areas of Europe. The most costly spice used in the world and is used for centuries to cook and for medicinal reasons. It's an incredible anti-aging component due to its richness in carotenoids and antioxidants: beta carotene, lycopene, and crocetin.

Orange is a fruit that has many advantages for our bodies:

It helps reduce inflammation.

Relaxes nervous and muscular spasms

This inhibits the growth of microbes and helps disinfect wounds

Conclusion

It is essential to recognize that humans are not created for ever. It is, however, possible to avoid the inevitable and extend your life. You can also be beautiful and flawless throughout your lifetime if you are prepared to take proper care of your physical and mental health.

Keep in mind that no amount of synthetic products or chemicals will help you look younger and attractive for a long period of time. The majority of them are short-term solutions that are only effective for a brief period. If this time period is over These products can cause numerous side effects that could even ruin your natural beauty and cause you to appear more aged.

Therefore, it is essential to only use natural products. Natural products can not only help you look younger however, they can aid in maintaining your youthful appearance for many years. The book is packed with the most natural solutions that will help you appear young and attractive.

While the recipes and products in this publication are organic and safe for use however, it is important to consult your doctor prior to making use of any of these items. There is a chance that you have an unknown allergy that could be in response to any of these ingredients. Therefore, it is important to be extremely cautious.